PKD The Kidney
An Alkaline Diet Geared to Kidney Health PKD Polycystic Kidney

BY
DANEVAS LLC

PKD The Kidney

Copyright © 2012 Danevas

All rights reserved.

ISBN 978-152-1302-729

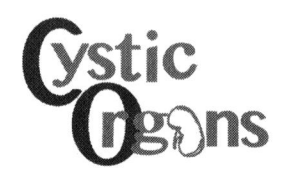

Cystic Organs

We are individuals with PKD. The following information is from empirical knowledge derived from individuals with cystic organ disease.

These are our experiences–a view from within a body riddled with cystic organs. Many of us have tried this diet.

As we age, this diet has been helpful to minimize PKD symptoms.

DEDICATION

This is dedicated to the fine doctors who have studied PKD. They have taken their time to research and understand PKD Polycystic Kidney Disease. This understanding is reflected in their treatment of us, giving many options for our medical management.

This is also dedicated to individuals with PKD Polycystic Kidney Disease who do not know where to turn, where to seek help, where to go once they have received the diagnosis of PKD.

Hormones, caffeine, chemicals (bleach, herbicides. pesticides, xenoestrogens, endocrine disruptors) all increase PKD symptoms. This book contains many detailed lists of items to be enjoyed and to be avoided for the maximum diminishing of PKD symptoms.

ACKNOWLEDGMENTS

I wish to thank those creative people whose contributions to this project have been invaluable~with the artwork, with the text, with the proof-reading, and with the layout.

FOREWORD

A single drop of water does not make a river.

~Author Unknown

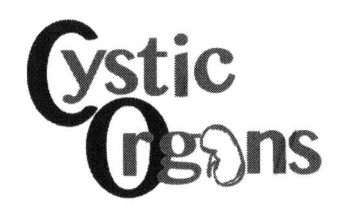

Cystic Organs

I wish to acknowledge those participants who have sent me their feedback with their willingness to try this diet and lifestyle changes. (Underlined words are links to the web.)

It has begun, this vast experiment that we are embarking on together. We have opened the doorway toward health.

TABLE OF CONTENTS

PKD The Kidney   1
An Alkaline Diet Geared to Kidney Health PKD Polycystic Kidney   1
DEDICATION   3
ACKNOWLEDGMENTS   4
FOREWORD   5
1. ABOUT PKD DIET   7
2. SUMMARY PKD DIET 13
3. TESTING ALKALINITY   16
4. NEUTRAL PROTEIN 18
5. SALT 20
6. WATER   22
7. DNA 25
8. BLOOD PRESSURE   26
9. ENJOY WITH PKD   28
10. ENJOY ANIMAL PROTEINS   76
11 ENJOY HERBS   77
12. ENJOY THESE GRAINS   83
13. USEFUL CHEMICALS 94
14. USEFUL VEGETABLES   100
15. USEFUL FRUITS   108
16. USEFUL SWEETENERS   113
17. BETTER PROTEIN CHOICES   114
18. HELPS WITH PKD   117
19. PKD CLINICAL TRIALS   118
20. AVOID ITEMS WITH PKD   120
21. AVOID ANIMAL PROTEINS 170
22. AVOID HERBS   179
24. AVOID GRAINS 187
25. AVOID DRINKS 195
26. AVOID CHEMICALS   202
27. AVOID VEGETABLES 219
28. AVOID FRUITS 224
29. AVOID SWEETENERS 227
30. EVERYONE TO AVOID   231
31. MENU   232
32. HELPFUL WEBSITES 238
33. DERMATOLOGY SYMPTOMS   239
34. ALKALINE CLINICAL TRIALS   241
35. THE FUTURE   244

1. ABOUT PKD DIET

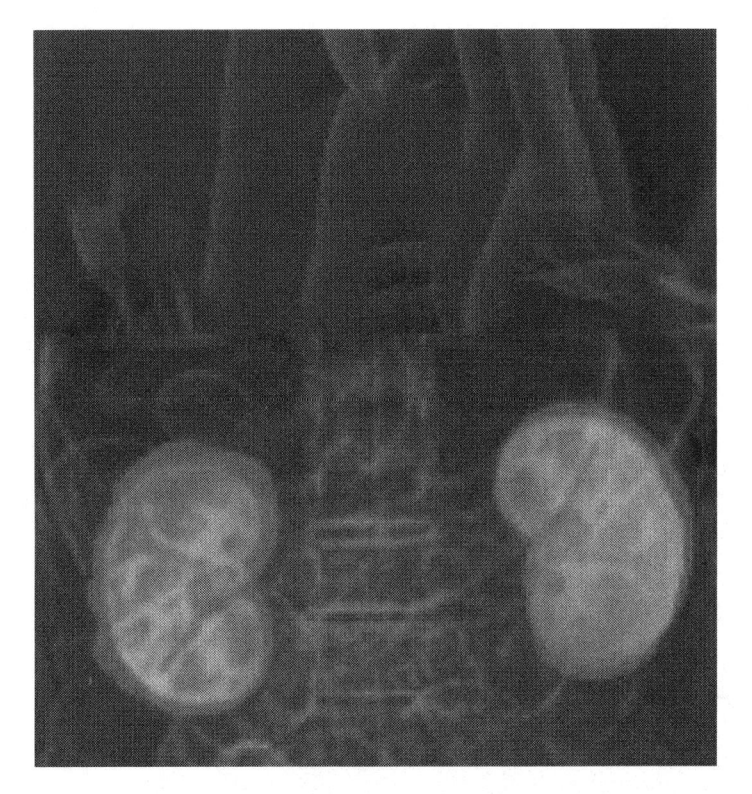

Plant based alkaline diet

Neutral Protein 0.6 grams/kg

1200 mg sodium

3 liters of water or 2x output

Low fat

Food restriction

The above diet is what some with PKD Polycystic Kidney Disease have tried. By making the switch to an alkaline vegan diet, cooking all foods yourself, without using canned, bottled or prepared substances, this greatly influences your body to become healthier.

Couple this with carefully choosing locally grown, non-GMO (non genetically engineered) produce, that is in season and purchased at its peak of ripeness can also positively influence the health polycystic kidney health.

If you have the ability or the inclination to grow your own fruits and vegetables, this too has many added benefits. Some mass produced foods (i.e., vegetables, chicken, etc.) are dipped in a bleach bath before coming to market or vegetables can be picked firm and green or grown especially to be transported instead of for its taste or nutritional content.

Other animal proteins have questionable processes performed. Learn more about this through viewing these interesting food documentaries and books:

    Food, Inc.
    Super Size Me
    Food Revolution LA
    The China Study
    No Happy Cows
    Forks Over Knives
    Best Diet

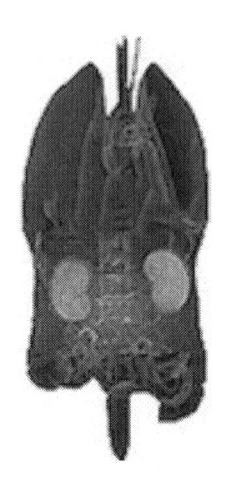

Some have gone as far as trying to eat a raw food diet of fruits and vegetables coupled with the avoids and enjoy list of foods from this diet. This raw food diet is said to be lowest in inflammation. Inflammation, according to the late Dr. Grantham, is what triggers cyst growth. A gluten free diet is also lower in inflammation. Avoiding nightshade plants (tomatoes, potatoes, peppers, eggplant) decreases inflammation.

By incorporating dietary and lifestyle changes many have successfully diminished countless PKD Polycystic Kidney Disease symptoms, including painful events and bloating episodes. Some have experienced an increase in energy; some have halted PKD kidney growth; some have experienced a lowering of blood pressure; eventually being able to eliminate all medication and there are also a lucky few who have noticed an improvement in their kidney functioning as they age. Most with PKD see a decline in kidney functioning around age 50.

Polycystic Kidney Disease PKD is an inherited disease that causes the normally smooth kidney tissue to enlarge and contain within it numerous fluid filled balloon like cysts. PKD cysts multiply and replace normal functioning kidney cells. With this change in the kidney structure, one result can be high blood pressure, spilling protein in the urine, and diminished kidney functioning. Oftentimes dialysis and kidney transplant are sought after treatments in the later years. Traditionally, symptoms increase with age; whereas those on this diet have discovered an overall bettering of their sense of well-being and a diminishing of symptoms.

We are not seeking a cure for Polycystic Kidney Disease. We are collectively asking the answer to the following question,

"How can we maintain the health of our polycystic organs and our transplanted organs?"

PKD diet is one possibility to try to see if it might work as well as it has for some of us. with PKD Polycystic Kidney Disease. Individual health issues are known by you. and your doctor. These pages are only meant as guides, as suggestions for you to try to incorporate.

Alkaline foods generally are fruits and vegetables–enjoy these freely. Acidic foods are animal proteins–these are limited. There are a few exceptions. Generally the sweeter the taste of a raw fruit or vegetable, the more alkaline producing it is. Continue to avoid nightshade plants and those that are high in oxalic acids. This can lead to kidney stones. Starfruit is a known high oxalic food. Avoid starfruit as it can lead to kidney demise.

Besides animal proteins causing acidity, other acid producing culprits are concentrated sugars and alcohols. Alcohol ferments are extremely harmful for PKD. These are ferments from wine, alcohol, yeasted baked goods. A bread baked by oneself without any additional yeast, seems to squelch symptoms.

Thus far, through self-testing, a usable alkaline sweetener could be tupelo honey or the addition of dried fruits, bananas, dates, raisins, or cinnamon. These additions lend sweetness to a dish. Recipe inspirations can be found at *http://www.PKDrecipes.com*. Foods prepared with other concentrated sugars have been known to cause urinary pH to register acidic (pH 5), raise serum cholesterol, create mood swings, increase cystic organ symptoms, and oftentimes trigger the onset of a painful headache even a migraine.

If one can eliminate animal proteins, and continue to obtain a daily intake of essential amino acids and essential fatty acids, this is better for polycystic organ health. Essential fatty acids are those needed by the body each day. Some vegetable food sources of essential fatty acids are chia, hempseed, and purslane.

Vegetables that contain sulfurins or cruciferous vegetables, typically contain many of the essential amino acids to be consumed daily: i.e., broccoli, Brussel sprouts, cabbage, turnips, or rutabagas. Juicing of these vegetables also helps increase the amount of nutrients and essential amino acids absorbed. Young cereal grasses can contribute an amino acid rich juice. The molecule for heme from hemoglobin, looks very similar to the spelt grass juice molecule. Drinking cereal grass juices may help correct anemia.

Other sources of proteins are grains, nuts, seeds, legumes, and beans, all soaked to diminish their phytic acid content. Spelt has the highest protein source of all the grains and lowest amount of phytic acid. Whereas wheat has been modified by commercial farming techniques and contains the highest amount of phytic acid of all the grains.

Sprouts, especially sprouted grains, are high in amino acids. Researchers discovered that broccoli sprouts or DIMs contains more than 50x the nutrients of a whole plant. Sprouting of seeds helps to diminish phytates or phytic acid within a food. Phytates maybe beneficial for some but not for those with PKD. If one is gluten intolerant, some useful grains are arrowroot, tapioca flour, coconut flour, almond flour, bean flour, sunchoke flour.

Soak grains, nuts, seeds, beans in water before eating thus diminishing the phytic acid. This has been developed by the plant to assure it will grow in the wild. Sprouting seeds also works! The seed coats itself with phytic acid so if swallowed, the person or animal eliminates the seed or the germ untouched. It surrounds itself with minerals from the body, to assure that the seed will sprout. If it the seed is sprouted this squelches the phytate activity. Soaking beans and lentils also aids their digestibility and decreases the amount of gas produced.

Another possibility is for one to limit the daily intake of animal proteins to three ounces or less; no more often than two or three times a week. The size of a deck of cards corresponds to about three ounces of fish. one dice is the equivalent of one ounce of cheese.

With PKD Polycystic Kidney Disease, eating animal proteins can cause many of us to spill proteins in our urine, an early sign of an impending decrease in kidney functioning. This eventually leads to declining kidney functioning. Through this PKD dietary modifications many have been able to join the 40% of individuals with PKD who never need dialysis or transplant.

Researchers have also discovered a low fat diet and a food restricted diet is helpful for the expression of PKD Polycystic Kidney Disease. This has been shown in the animal model only. Human clinical trials are yet to begin.

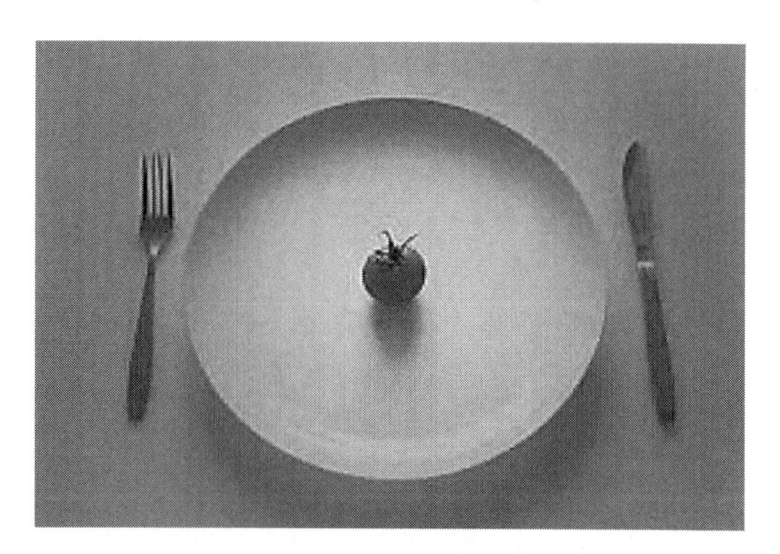

2. SUMMARY PKD DIET

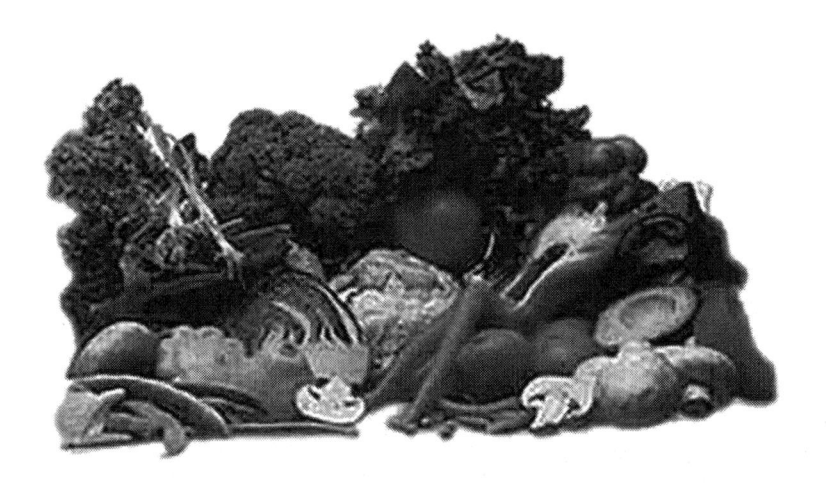

Here is a simpler form of the diet.
Below is a general summary of this PKD diet.

Foods to Avoid
The following foods should not be eaten for the PKD Diet to be effective.
- Avoid meat, poultry, fish and eggs~anything with a belly button, a face, a mother.
- Dairy products such as butter, cheese, cream, ice cream, yogurt, milk and skimmed milk.
- Oils: Limit to one ounce per day.
- Refined grains: Avoid White rice, *enriched* wheat flour found in pastas, yeasted breads, yeasted baked goods, yeasted bagels. In addition to wheat, avoid cheerios and flaxseed.
- Nuts: Heart disease Individuals should avoid nuts.
- Concentrated sugars: avoid table sugar, high fructose corn syrup, agave, coconut sugar, honey, (except tupelo honey, which is fine).

Foods That Are Allowed

- Vegetables - Except for nightshade plants, high oxalate vegetables, celery, GMO vegetables, caffeine containing vegetables. If you are a cardiac patient avocados are high n fat. Those that do not have heart disease may eat avocados.
- Legumes - Beans, peas, lentils, seeds soak to ↓ phytates. No soy.
- Whole Spelt, Rye, Rice (caution rice ↑ in arsenic). No wheat or yeast,
- Fruit, Any except no high oxalate fruits or nightshade fruits, such as rhubarb, sugar cane, mountain apples, noni, plums, strawberries, starfruit, prunes, whole cranberries, blueberries,
- Beverages PKD diet allows the following beverages: Water, seltzer water, almond or cashew milk with no-fat or added sugar. Hibiscus tea, chamomile tea, veronica tea, roasted grain beverages.

Supplements

- Vitamin B12 - 1000 mcg (micrograms) daily.
- Calcium - People over 50 should take 1000 milligrams daily, over 60 take 1200 mg daily or Vitamin K (if prescribed) or chelated calcium,
- Vitamin D - Those over 50 should take 500 IU daily.
- Omega Fatty Acids One hempseed tablet each day.
- Turmeric
- N Acetyl Choline (check with your doctor).
- Zinc, Folic Acid (if over 65)
* Water

Laboratory Test

- Total blood cholesterol should be 150mg/dL or less.
- LDL levels 80mg/dL or lower.
- GFR

- DEXA bone scan, + later spine x-ray, EKG, CXR
- Kidney function tests
- Liver function tests
- Mammogram (female >45)
- MRI size of kidneys & liver
- Head MRI rule out aneurysms
- Colonoscopy (with aging, once every 10 years) or Cologuard test

Researchers from Cornell University Have Discovered a Vegetarian Allele

- This might be one answer why some people have an easier time with veganism and others do not. This is tied to assimilating the fatty acids from plant based foods.

Only 5% of kidney cells become cysts but unlike liver cysts, kidney cysts replace functioning kidney tissue. That is, kidney cysts no longer function as true kidney tissue.

3. TESTING ALKALINITY

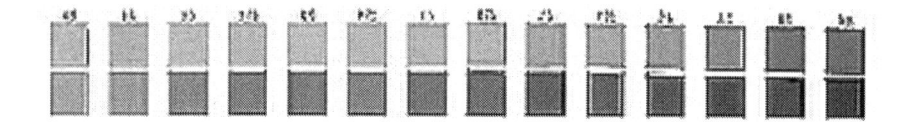

Test alkalinity at night just before bed

- *Plant based alkaline diet*

Using nitrazine paper, a dipstick, or pH paper on a roll (Vivid with a range of 5.5 - 8.0) self-testing of urinary pH is possible.

To test urinary pH: Do so at night, the last thing before going to sleep–

Tear a piece of pH paper and pass the torn paper strip through your urine stream. Read and compare the color change against the provided chart to determine your urinary pH.

Another method is to urinate into a disposable cup and dip pH nitrazine paper into the urine. If using pH paper on a roll is more to your liking, this is stocked by Micro essential labs.

Micro Essential
   https://goo.gl/YC6hdn
lab goods includes the most commonly requested roll which is **#067**. It has a range of 5.5 to 8.0 - 3 roll refills.

Amazon also carries the pH tape.
https://amzn.to/2GfxZOX

Testing pH dipsticks from pHion
https://amzn.to/2GdmlEb

Micro Essential

Testing dipsticks are thought to be easier to read.

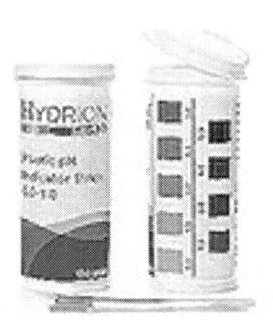

You can change the health of your cystic organs. It is possible. You will always have the PKD Polycystic Kidney Disease gene but how it manifests within your body is something you can change, Individuals with PKD Polycystic Kidney Disease normally have acidic urine. This contributes to elevations in uric acid. 24% of individuals with PKD have full blown gout. Acidic urine can raise uric acid. High uric acid can expand into gout symptoms. Little crystals get stuck in the joints causing pain. This can contribute to kidney stone formation. By decreasing oxalates, purine foods, eating alkaline, lowering blood pressure, lowering proteinuria, eating less protein foods, eating less salt and drinking loads of water, this can result in PKD Polycystic Kidney Disease symptoms being kept under control.

A long PKD Medical article
[http://www.pkdiet.com/pdf/PKD.pdf]
explains about PKD Polycystic Kidney Disease.

4. NEUTRAL PROTEIN

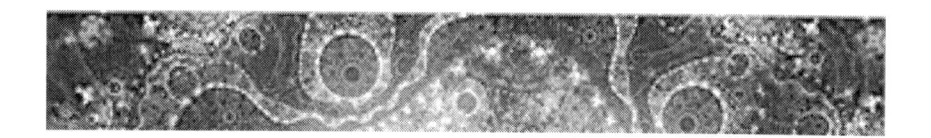

Test Between Doctor's Visits

- *Neutral Protein 0.6 grams/kg*

Neutral protein is achieved when the amount of protein eaten daily is equal to the amount that comes out, called a neutral balance. Eating extra protein puts weight on plus it unnecessarily increases the burden of the workload on PKD kidneys. This can cause spillage of protein in the urine, an early sign of decreasing kidney functioning. Neutral protein is 0.6 grams of protein per kilogram of body weight. Eating a neutral amount of protein helps PKD cystic kidneys remain healthier by diminishing proteinuria and allowing cystic kidneys to more readily eliminate any toxins and acids from the body. This in turn keeps a PKD cystic kidneys healthy. Eating proteins changes the stomach pH toward acidic. Calculate Your Neutral Protein:

NEUTRAL PROTEIN
Convert your body weight from pounds to kg.
If one weighs 110 pounds, divide 110 by 2.2 = 50 kg.
If one weighs 176 pounds, divide 176 by 2.2 = 80 kg.

Multiply your kg of body weight by 0.6 grams of protein.
For a 110 pound person: multiply 50 kg by 0.6 =
30 grams of protein per day.

For a 176 pound person: multiply 80 kg by 0.6 =
48 grams of protein per day

At the very minimum, limit animal protein to three ounces or less per day and no more often than two or three times a week. A protein chart,

[http://www.polycystic-kidneydisease.com/html/pkd_loprochart.html]

prepared by a fellow PKD'r contains some protein values for certain food items.

Later in this book a list of better protein choices *(chapter 17)* are given. If one cannot make the switch totally to plants then better animal proteins are listed. These protein choices are better for cystic disease organs. Fish is too high in pesticides concentrated in the oceans' runoff from farms and corporations. If one enjoys cheese there are plant based cheeses available. If not, a soft white dairy cheese is preferable to a hard dry orange cheese.

5. SALT

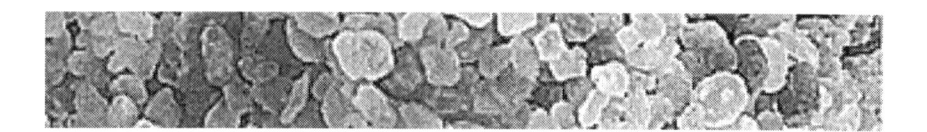

↓ Salt Lowers Blood Pressure

- *1200 mg Sodium*

One-eighth teaspoon of salt is equivalent to 1200 mg of sodium. Due to the hidden salt in many prepared foods cooking your own food without salt goes a long way toward staying on a 1200 mg sodium diet.

Table salt contains aluminum to make it free flowing. Higher amounts of aluminum have been found on autopsy in the brains of individuals with dementia and Alzheimer's.

Instead try grinding fresh Himalayan pink crystal salt,

[http://www.pkdiet.com/diet_Himalayansalt.php]

Continue to limit Himalayan salt to one-eighth teaspoon per day. If permitted, try 2-5 drops of solé in a full glass of water daily.

[http://www.pkdrecipes.com/?p=1516]

Take a few drops of solé in the morning with a full glass of water. For most this seems to help PKD Polycystic Kidney Disease symptoms. Others have noted that taking solé can raise their blood pressure. Or that salt in the water causes swelling,

A few notes from a friend on solé:

[http://www.pkdiet.com/diet_soleMore.php#notes]

As we age by using Himalayan salt exclusively, we maintain the exact same proportions of minerals from the chemical scale that are needed by the body. By using Himalayan salt the amount of aluminum in our brains is decreased, hopefully helping prevent dementia as we age,

In Hawaii, researchers have discovered that those populations eating more soy tofu, more soy products~ these individuals go much more quickly toward dementia as they age. This is thought to be due to the aluminum pipes used in the commercial preparation of soy products. In other cases it has been due to the genetically modified soy bean, prominent in Hawaii.

6. WATER

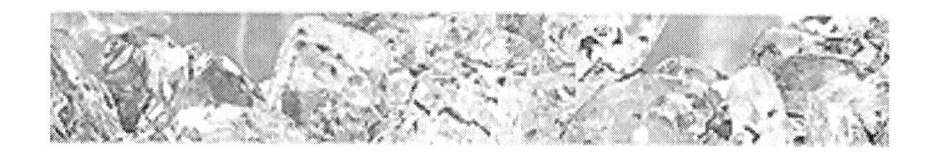

Shut down vasopressin

- *4 liters of water or 2x output*

If permitted, drink enough water to suppress vasopressin release. This is twice urinary output or approximately 4 liters of water per day (4 quarts). Vasopressin triggers cyst growth. Decreased cyst growth slows down PKD Polycystic Kidney Disease size, development, and symptoms.

A Low-Osmolar Diet study was undertaken at Tufts University in the USA. Four liters was the required amount of water to shut down vasopressin, a protein involved in cyst growth.
 https://www.ncbi.nlm.nih.gov/pubmed/27663039

Researchers have concluded that drinking 4 liters of water in addition to other liquids (herbal tea, juice, etc.), will shut down vasopressin, a protein the signals cyst growth. A liter of water is approximately equal to a quart.

40% of those with PKD never require dialysis or transplant. Sometimes these are those who have inherited PKD2, the less aggressive form of PKD Polycystic Kidney Disease. We wish to be included amongst those 40%.

A few things best avoided with Polycystic Kidney Disease:

Aspirin, Tylenol®, Paracetamol, Acetaminophen

Advil, NSAIDs, Ibuprofen

Animal proteins limit to no more than 3 ounces/day: 2-3 times/week

Bleach: Clorox®, bleach cleansers, chicken dipped in bleach, carrots dipped in bleach

<u>Caffeine</u>: chocolate, coffee, tea, cola, soda, pop

Chlorine, chloride, carbon tetrachloride, plastic BPA

Dichloroacetate DCA, sometimes added to city tap water

Lithium

Nightshade plants, high in oxalates

Phenacetin (Howard Hughes died from this).

Starfruit

Sodium bicarbonate, baking soda, can increase kidney stone formation, 20% higher incidence with PKD

Sugar, concentrated sugars

Tea: black, green, white, de-caffeinated, as well as certain herb teas

For the best city tap water
https://www.ewg.org/tapwater/#.WuuZ9i-ZORe
Key in your zip code or try this pdf
http://www.pkdiet.com/pdf/Top%2010%20Tap%20Water%20Cities.pdf

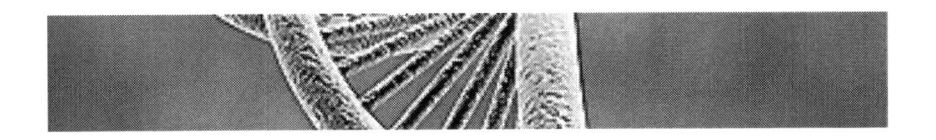

7. DNA

Shut down vasopressin
• Protect the Integrity of Your DNA

Use all means possible to protect the integrity of your DNA; squelching the second hit inheritance.

[http://www.pkdiet.com/pkd2hit.php]

We each have inherited the gene for PKD Polycystic Kidney Disease, but how it manifests in each of us is different, including how others within families may manifest PKD. What causes this? The same things that cause cancers to manifest in a body. How to prevent this? Protect your own DNA.

Try DIMs (broccoli sprouts), Turmeric (curcumin~better absorption is achieved with Black Pepper), Milk thistle are a few items that protect your own DNA. Water or staying well hydrated is a great DNA protector keeping your cells plumped, protecting the DNA further.

Avoid acrylamide. It is present in grains, potatoes, corn, that are heated to 248°, this forms acrylamide. To decrease acrylamide, try boiling your vegetables, then baking them. If you find your self exposed to acrylamide, check with your doctor and with his to her blessing, take N-Acetyl Cysteine which also protects your DNA.

8. BLOOD PRESSURE

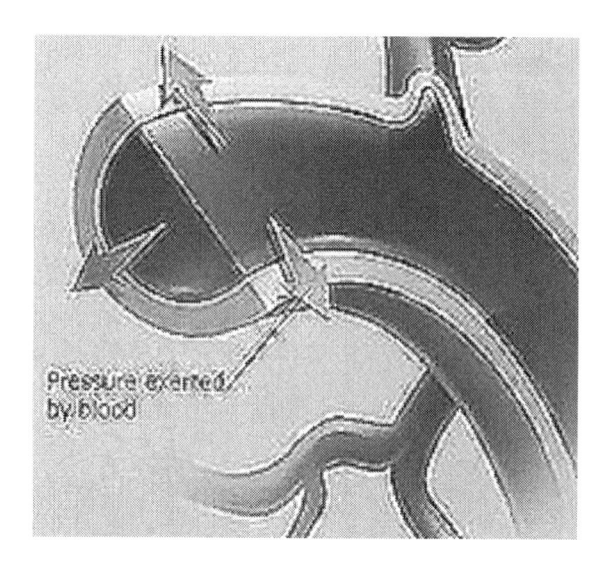

Test Blood Pressure upon awakening
- *Keep Tightly Controlled Blood Pressure*

Check your PKD blood pressure daily~in the morning when PKD blood pressure is highest. Be sure it stays between 119/79. If it is out of this range, contact your physician and get help in maintaining a low blood pressure. Keeping your blood pressure tightly controlled near 119/79 goes a long way toward preventing kidney decline. Normally others blood pressure (without PKD) is higher in the evening,
Other things to do for Blood Pressure:
Avoid allergic foods: soy, dairy, wheat, sesame seeds.
Take daily walks.

Avoid caffeine.

For a more complete discussion try this website:
http://www.pkdiet.com/pkdBP.php

Get a blood pressure device and have it calibrated at each doctor's visit. There are certain blood pressure medications better for PKD'rs than others, ACE and ACEi. These not only lower blood pressure but also decrease proteinuria and increase blood flow to the kidneys.

If your blood pressure is normal (100/70 - 110/60 - 120/80), maintain this blood pressure by continuing to limit salt. Brown rice (rinse frequently to diminish arsenic) and vegetables is good starting point. Go for daily gentle walks. Keep a lower body weight. Eat mostly vegetables. Avoid the top ten allergic foods as well as any food allergies. Get sufficient rest, drink plenty of water, eliminate caffeine including even all decaffeinated drinks, and stay warm.

If you do not have the means to purchase a blood pressure cuff then take your own blood pressure at pharmacies, drug stores, warehouse stores wherever you there is a public blood pressure machine.
There is a machine called RESperate

[https://www.resperate.com]

that lowers blood pressure. Check with your doctor.

There is also another device called DiaDens-Cardio-2

[http://www.denas-store.com/diadens-cardio.html]

that lowers blood pressure. Ask your doctor if either of these devices might be appropriate for you.

9. ENJOY WITH PKD

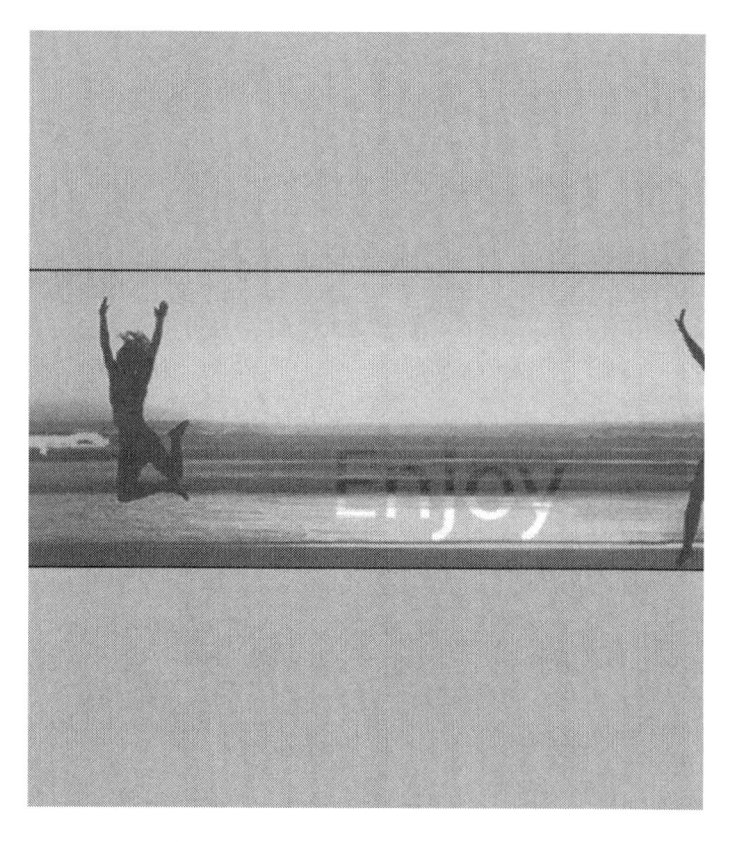

To follow are a list of items to be enjoyed. We know that these are to be enjoyed as this list of items does not seem to increase symptoms from PKD. See this enjoy list of items.

We with PKD have spent our time testing each item daily by measuring our abdominal girth at the same time at the same point and we have each made note if we experienced any pain or girth changes or kidney changes. To read further about these items try:

AlkalineDiet.com/enjoy.html or PKDiet.com/foods.php

PKDiet.com/foods_herbs.php or PKDiet.com/foods_otc.php

ENJOY WITH PKD

ACE

ACEi caution elderly

Acerola

Acorn squash

Adzuki beans

Agaricus bisporus (mushroom)

Albumin

Alkalinity

All fruit spread

Allium

Almond butter

Almond milk (√ no carrageenan)

Almond milk ice cream (√ no carrageenan)

Almond oil

ENJOY WITH PKD

Almond yogurt(√ no carrageenan)

Almond yogurt smoothie (√ no carrageenan)

Almonds / Amaranth

Amino acids to ↑ kidney functioning

Anasazi beans

Anti-inflammatory foods / Antibiotics when needed

Anutra / Aojiru

Apollinaris water/ Apple

Apple banana

Apple cider Ø sugar

Apple concentrate as sweetener

Apple juice fresh

Apple sauce

Apple sweet

ENJOY WITH PKD

Apricot

Apricot juice

ARB angiotensin receptor site blockers

Arginex/ Aronia / Aronia juice / Aronia melanocarpa

Arrowroot   treatment poisoned arrow wound

Artichoke

Artichoke flour

Artichoke leaf

Artichokes globe

Artichokes Jerusalem

Artichokes sunchoke girasola 👍

Artocarpus altilis (breadfruit) / Arugula

Asparagus (urine will become acidic)

Asteraceae

ENJOY WITH PKD

Avocado

Avocado oil

Baby spring greens / Badoit water

Bamboo shoots

Banana

Baps spelt

Barley

Barley milk Ø carrageenan sugar

Barley grass / Barley grass juice

Barley powder

Bartlett pear

Bay leaf

Bean flour

Bean sprout noodles

ENJOY WITH PKD
Bean sprouts
Bean threads vermicelli
Beans soak all
Beans string, snap
Beef tea / Beef consommé / Beef restoran distilled
Beet tops ↑ oxalates
Beetroot
Beets / beet juice
Bellis perennis
Bentonite clay
Berry
Berry juice
Besan flour
Bilberry juice

ENJOY WITH PKD
Bing cherry juice
Bing cherries
Biodynamic
Bio magnet pairs / Biotin B7
Bitter melon
Black beans
Black currants
Black eyed peas
Black lentils
Black raspberry
Black rice
Black turtle beans
Blackberry
Blackberry juice

ENJOY WITH PKD
Blue Zones
Blueberry juice
Bok choy
Bon ami
Borax laundry booster
Boron / Borsec water
Boysenberry
Brassica
Brazil nuts caution aflatoxin
Bread Ø yeast or wheat
Breadfruit/ Breadnut
Breast milk
Brisdelle (paroxetine) wait / Broad beans
Broccoli

ENJOY WITH PKD

Broccoli DIMs 👍

Broccoli rabe

Broccoli sprouts

Brown lentils

Brown rice

Brown rice noodles

Brussels sprouts

Bubble water

Buckwheat

Buckwheat noodles

Buckwheat sprouts

Buddha's hand

Burdock oil

Burdock root

ENJOY WITH PKD

Butter beans soak

Button mushrooms

Cabbage

Cabbage Chinese

Cabbage juice

Cabbage red

Cabbage savoy

Caf-lib / Cafix /Calamansi

Calcium citrate

Calcium vegan foods

Cannabidiol

Cannellini beans soak

Cantaloupe local (transported develops fungus)

Cantharellus cibarius (chanterelle)

ENJOY WITH PKD
Caraway seeds
Cardoon
Caro / Carob
Carrot juice fresh
Carrots
Carum carvi (caraway) / Casaba melon
Cashews
Cassava (manioc, yuca root, tapioca)
Cauliflower
CBD (cannabidiol)
Celeriac
Cellophane noodles
Cèpes mushrooms
Cereal grass juice

ENJOY WITH PKD
Chamomile 👍
Chamomile tea
Channa flour
Chanterelle mushrooms
Chard / Charlotte's web
Chateldon water
Chayote squash
Cherimoya
Cherry / Cherry juice
Cherry Montmorency
Cherry sour / Cherry sour juice
Chestnut
Chia / Chia drink
Chia oil / Chia oil capsules

ENJOY WITH PKD
Chia seeds
Chickpea / Chickpea flour
Chico
Chicory
Chinese cabbage
Chinese peas
Chives
Chokeberry juice
Cilantro
Cinnamon
Citrus fruits / Citrus juice fresh
Clear noodles
Clementine
Clementine juice fresh

ENJOY WITH PKD
Club soda / Cobalamin
Coconut aminos / Coconut butter
Coconut especially young coconut spoon meat
Coconut flour / Coconut milk
Coconut milk ice cream
Coconut water / Coenzyme Q10
Coffee alternatives
Colgate wisp mini Toothbrush
Collard greens
Colocasia esculenta (taro)
CoQ10
Corn bread organic Ø wheat Ø sugar Ø GMO
Corn meal organic
Corn organic Ø GMO

ENJOY WITH PKD

Corn salad nüssli mache

Corn tortillas organic

Cranberry juice avoid whole fruit

Creasy greens

Crêpes made with buckwheat

Crimini

Crookneck squash

Cruciferous vegetables

Cucumber peel the skin

Cucumber juice

Cumin

Curcumin

Currants

Curry leaf

ENJOY WITH PKD
Custard apple
Daikon radish
Daisy
Daiya
Dal
Dasheen araimo (taro)
Date sugar
Dates
Deadnettle
Delicata squash
DIMs (broccoli sprouts) 👍
Dinkel
Donut peaches
Dr. Collins Restore toothpaste

ENJOY WITH PKD

Dragon fruit

Dried fruit

Drumstick plant 👍

Dryland cress

Durian

Ecoplasts

Eddoes root

Edible flowers / Einkorn (spelt)

Elderberry juice

Elderberry syrup / Emmer (farro)

Emu oil

Endive chicory

English peas / Erythropoietin

Escarole

ENJOY WITH PKD

Farro

Fava soak peel beans

Ferrarelle water

Figs 👍 dried fresh

Flageolets / Floradix

Fluoride carrageenan free toothpaste

Food restricted / Forbidden rice

Fresca Chia

Fruit / Fruit concentrate

Fuji apples

Fuzzy toothbrush

GABA rice

Gabi taro

Gac, a tropical fruit

ENJOY WITH PKD

Gala apples

Galangal

Garbanzo beans chick peas

Garbanzo flour

Garlic / Garlic oil

Gelatin

Gerolsteiner water

Ghassoul

Girasola

Globe artichoke

Gobi

Golden delicious apple

Golden raspberry

Gooseberry

ENJOY WITH PKD
Grain beverage barley brew
Grain beverage barley cup
Grain beverage cafix
Grain beverage caro
Grain beverage carob powder
Grain beverage inka
Grain beverage java herb uncoffee
Grain beverage kara kara
Grain beverage organic instant grain / Oshawa coffee
Grain beverage pero
Grain beverage prewetts chicory
Grain beverage roma
Grain beverage spelt kaffee
Grain beverage teeccino

ENJOY WITH PKD

Grain beverage yorzo

Gram flour

Grape juice

Grape juice concentrate

Grape seed

Grape seed extract

Grapefruit caution

Grapefruit juice caution

Grapes

Gravenstein apple

Great northern bean

Green brown lentils

Green juices

Greens collard

ENJOY WITH PKD

Greens leafy / Greens leafy kale

Greens mustard

Greens purslane

Grits organic

Groats

Guava

Gumbo file powder

H2 blockers (if needed)

Haricots verts / Harmless Harvest coconut water

Hazelnut milk (√ no carrageenan)

Hearts of palm

Helianthus tuberosus

Hempseed

Hempseed butter

ENJOY WITH PKD
Hempseed milk
Hempseed oil
Hempseed oil capsules
Herb tea Bamboo
Herb tea blood orange
Herb tea burdock root
Herb tea chamomile
Herb tea chamomile citrus
Herb tea hibiscus ↓BP
Herb tea lemon balm
Herb tea lemon thyme
Herb tea lemon water 👍
Herb tea lemongrass
Herb Tea lime leaf

ENJOY WITH PKD

Herb Tea linden flower

Herb tea linden flower leaves

Herb tea milk thistle

Herb tea milk thistle sylimarin

Herb tea mint magic

Herb tea nettle leaf

Herb tea peppermint

Herb tea rose hips

Herb tea saffron 👍

Herb tea silymarin 👍

Herb tea soba

Herb tea speedwell

Herb tea sugar cookie sleigh ride

Herb tea thyme

ENJOY WITH PKD
Herb tea tilleul
Herb tea veronica 👍
Herb tea watermelon seed
Hibiscus 👍
Himalayan pink salt
Honeydew melon
Honeydew melon juice
Huckleberry juice
Iron foods ↑ iron
Inositol
Injera
Iron innate response (when prescribed)
Iskiate
Jackfruit

ENJOY WITH PKD

Jerusalem artichoke 👍

Jicama

Kabocha squash

Kale

Kale juice

Kamut

Kidney beans

Kiwi

Klettenwurzel haar oil

Kohlrabi

Komatsuna

Krachai

Kumquat

Lamb's lettuce, mache lettuce

ENJOY WITH PKD
Lamium purpureum
Land cress
Langka
Lanreotide
Leafy greens
Leeks
Lemon 👍
Lemon balm
Lemon egg
Lemon hot
Lemon juice freshly squeezed 👍
Lemon thyme
Lemonade Ø sugar
Lemongrass

ENJOY WITH PKD
Lemons Meyer
Lentils soaked
Lettuce butter
Lettuce curly leaf
Lettuce mache, lamb's lettuce
Lettuce oak leaf
Lettuce romaine
Leucine
Lilikoi
Lima beans butter beans
Lime
Lime flower tea
Lime juice
Lime leaf

ENJOY WITH PKD
Linden flower
Linden flower tea
Liver useful
Long bean threads
Loquat
Lotus root
Low fat
Lungkow vermicelli
Lutein
Lycopene
Mache lettuce
Magnesium citrate (if OK)
Magnesium oil (if OK)
Magnet pairs

ENJOY WITH PKD

Malunggay leaves

Malungai

Mandarins

Mango

Mangosteen

Manihot esculenta

Manikara zapota sapodilla (chico)

Manioc cassava yuca

Manuka bush

Manuka honey

Marjoram

Marrow beans

Marshmallow herb

Masa maiz

ENJOY WITH PKD
Melissa cream
Melissa Extract Non-Aclcoholic
Melon juice
Melon smooth skinned 👍
Menoquinone Ø Soy
Meso-zeaxanthin
Meyer lemon
Milk thistle silymarin
Mineral water
Mint ↑ GERD
Miracle berry / Miraculin
Mixed wild greens
Mizuna / Mochi brown rice
Montmorency cherry / Morchella

ENJOY WITH PKD
Morels
Moringa oleifera
Moroccan red clay
Mother's milk
Mulberry juice
Mung bean noodles
Mung bean sprouts
Mung bean
Murungai
Murungai leaves 👍
Mushrooms edible
Mustard greens
Mustard seed
Myrtle

ENJOY WITH PKD
Napa
Naringenin 👍
Nasturtiums
Natto Ø soy
Nattokinase Ø Soy
Naval oranges / Navy beans
Nectarines
Nettle ↓ uric acid
Nettle extract non alcoholic 👍
Niaxium
NMN Nictinamide Mononucleaotide
Northern beans / Nüssli (mache)
Nüssli (mache)
O3 Pure Ozone Laundry

ENJOY WITH PKD
Oak leaf lettuce
Oat milk (√ no carrageenan)
Oats
Octreotide
Oil almond / Oil hemp seed oil
Okinawan sweet potato
Okra
Olive caution with salt
Olive oil limit 1 ounce/day
Olive leaf
Omeprazole / Onions
Opo
Orange
Orange juice freshly squeezed

ENJOY WITH PKD
Orange lentils
Oregano ↓ candidiasis
Oyster plant
Pak choi
Pantoprazole / Papaya
Papaya juice fresh pressed
Paroxetine
Parsnip
Pasireotide (wait)
Passion fruit
Pasta spelt, kamut, brown rice, artichoke
Pasta whole grains Ø wheat
Paw paw
Pea

ENJOY WITH PKD
Peach
Peach smoothies Ø sugar
Pear
Pecans
Pellegrino water
Peppermint
Pero
Perrier
Persimmon
Pineapple
Pineapple juice
Pink apples
Pinto bean
Pithaya

ENJOY WITH PKD

Plantain

Polenta organic

Pomelo

Popcorn organic ∅ salt

Porcini / Portobello mushrooms

Potassium citrate

Potatoes sweet

Potatoes sweet jewel

Potatoes sweet Okinawan / Prebiotics

Prilosec / Proteinuria ↓

Proton pump inhibitors possibly / Protonix

Pumpkin

Pumpkin seed oil

Purple archangel / Purslane / Pyridoxine

ENJOY WITH PKD
Queen Anne cherries
Quince
Quinoa soaked
Radish 👍
Radish sprouts
Rainier cherry / Raisin organic
Ramon seed
Ramps wild onions / Rapamycin
Rapini
Raspberry caution pregnancy
Raspberry leaf
Raw local produce
Raw unheated coconut water
Red banana / Red bean

ENJOY WITH PKD

Red cabbage / Red cabbage juice

Red currants / Red dead nettleRed kuru pumpkin

Red kuru pumpkin

Red lentils

Red onion

Red rice (not yeast) caution arsenic

Rhassoul clay

Rhizomes / Riboflavin

Rice crackers

Rice ice cream

Rice milk (√ no sugar, arsenic, carrageenan)

Roasted grain tea

Romaine lettuce

Rose hips

ENJOY WITH PKD

Rutabagas / Rutin

Rye

Rye bread Ø yeast

Rye crackers Ø yeast

Rye crisps Ø yeast

Saffron

Saffron tea

Sago root sago tapioca pearls

Salsify oyster plant goatsbeard

Salt Himalayan / Sambucol

Samsca (caution liver)

San Pellegrino water

Sandostatin LAR

Sapodilla (chico)

ENJOY WITH PKD
Sapote
Saturn peaches
Savoy cabbage
Scallions / Shallots
Shampoo Ø formaldehyde
Shampoo Ø methylisothiazoline MIT
Shampoo Ø methylpaprabens
Shampoo Ø parabens
Shampoo Ø phthalates
Shampoo Ø sodium lauryl sulfate
Shea butter / Shohl's / Slymarin
Slippery elm
Smooth skinned melons
Snap peas / Snow peas

ENJOY WITH PKD

Soba noodles Ø wheat /Soda water

Sodium citrate

Solé /Sour cherry/ Sour cherry juice

Speedwell

Spelt / Spelt bread Ø yeast 👍

Spelt crackers Ø yeast wheat flax

Spelt grass juice

Spelt pasta

Spelt stuffing / Spring onions

Spring water

Sprouts broccoli

Sprouts chickpea

Sprouts corn Ø GMO

Sprouts mung bean

ENJOY WITH PKD

Sprouts pea

Sprouts radish

Squash

Stem cells wait

Stinging nettle

String beans

Stuffing Ø wheat

Succotash

Summer savory

Sunchoke Jerusalem artichoke / Sunchoke flour 👍

Swedes

Sweet potato

Swiss chard / Sylmarin

Tangelo

ENJOY WITH PKD

Tangerine

Tangerine juice

Tannia root

Tapioca sago or cassava

Taro root / Taste Nirvana coconut water

Teff

Test alkalinity

Test blood pressure

Test proteinuria

Thai ginger

Thiamine

Thyme / Thyme tea

Tight blood pressure control

Tilleul

ENJOY WITH PKD
Tilleul tea
Tolvaptan caution liver
Truffle (fungus)
Tsamma juice
Tupelo
Tupelo honey
Turban squash
Turmeric 👍
Turnip
Turnip greens
Ube
Ugli fruit 👍
Urtica dioica
Vanilla bean / Vanilla powder

ENJOY WITH PKD

Vasopressin ↓ / Vegetable juice fresh

Vegan cream cheese/ Vegetable korma/ Vegetable pakora

Velikdenche / Veniafaxine (effexor)

Vermicelli clear

Veronica / Veronica tea 👍

Vitamin B1 / Vitamin B12

Vitamin B2 / Vitamin B6

Vitamin B7

Vitamin C

Vitamin D

Vitamin E

Vitamin K2 Ø soy (if prescribed)

Walnuts

Washing soda

ENJOY WITH PKD

Water

Water chestnuts

Watercress

Watermelon local

Watermelon juice 👍

Watermelon seed tea 👍

Wattwiller water

Wax beans

Welch onion scallions

Wheatgrass juice

White asparagus

White beans

White carrots / White mushrooms

White nectarines

ENJOY WITH PKD

White peaches

White radish / White yam

Whole grains organic Ø wheat

Wild onion ramps

Wild rice

Winter squash

Yams

Yellow currants / Yellow onions

Yellow squash

Yoga / Yuca

Zapota (chico) / Zeaxanthin / Zegerid

Zicoh coconut water / Zucchini (√ not GMO)

👍 especially useful

10. ENJOY ANIMAL PROTEINS

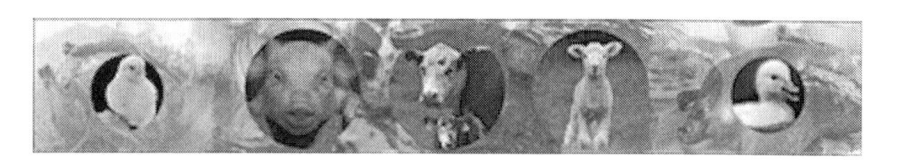

ENJOY ANIMAL PROTEINS
Beef consommé
Beef restoran
Beef distilled stock
Beef tea
Gelatin

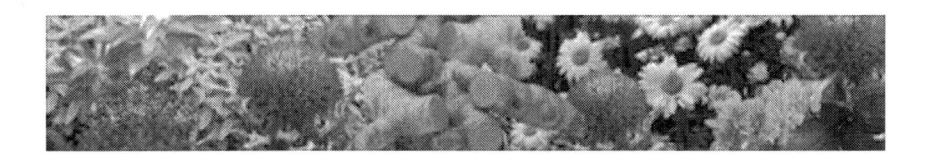

11 ENJOY HERBS

ENJOY HERBS
Allium sativum
Artichoke leaf
Asteraceae
Bay leaf
Bellis perennis
Breadnut
Cannabidiol
Caraway
Carcum carvi
CBD (cannabidiol)

ENJOY HERBS
Chamomile
Chives
Cilantro
Cinnamon ↑ GERD, helps regulate blood sugar
Cumin
Curry leaf
Elderberry
Galangal
Garlic
Gumbo file (non-carcinogenic)
Hempseed
Hibiscus ↓ Blood Pressure
Himalayan pink salt (Limit to an eighth teaspoon per day)

ENJOY HERBS
Garlic
Gumbo file (non-carcinogenic)
Hempseed
Hibiscus ↓ Blood Pressure
Himalayan pink salt (Limit to an eighth teaspoon per day)
Krachai
Lamium purpureum (purple dead nettle)
Lemon balm
Lemon thyme
Lemongrass
Lime leaf
Linden flower
Mallunggay leaves ↑ iron stores

ENJOY HERBS
Manuka
Marjoram
Marshmallow
Melissa
Milk thistle silymarin
Mint ↑ GERD
Moringa oleifera
Mustard seed
Myrtle
Nettle ↓ uric acid
Olive leaf
Oregano ↓ candidiasis
Peppermint ↑ GERD

ENJOY HERBS
Purple archangel (red deadnettle)
Ramon seed
Raspberry leaf caution pregnancy
Rose hip
Saffron ↓ BP
Saffron tea
Salt Himalayan (Limit to an eighth teaspoon per day)
Sambucol
Shea butter
Silymarin
Slippery elm
Solé
Speedwell

ENJOY HERBS
Stinging nettle
Summer savory
Thai ginger
Thyme
Tilleul
Tupelo
Turmeric
Urtica dioica
Vanilla bean
Vanilla powder
Velikdenche
Veronica
Watermelon seed

12. ENJOY THESE GRAINS

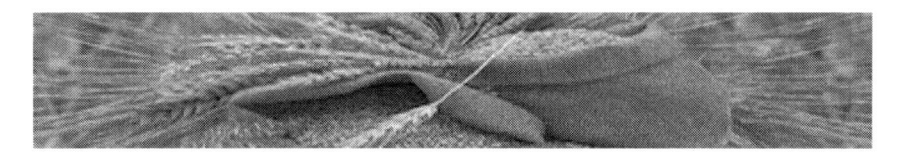

To ↓ Phytates, soak before preparing

USEFUL GRAINS, GRAINS, NUTS, SEEDS, BEANS LEGUMES
Adzuki bean
Almond butter
Almonds
Amaranth
Anasazi beans
Anutra
Arrowroot
Artichoke flour
Baps spelt

USEFUL GRAINS, GRAINS, NUTS, SEEDS, BEANS LEGUMES
Barley
Bean flour
Bean sprouts
Bean thread vermicelli
Beans soaked
Besan flour
Black bean
Black eyed peas
Black lentils
Black rice ~caution ↑ arsenic
Black turtle beans
Brazil nuts caution arsenic, selenium
Bread Ø wheat yeast

USEFUL GRAINS, GRAINS, NUTS, SEEDS, BEANS LEGUMES
Broad beans
Brown lentils
Brown rice caution arsenic
Brown rice noodles caution arsenic
Buckwheat
Buckwheat noodles
Butter beans
Cannellini beans
Carob
Cashews
Cassava, tapioca, yuca root, manioc
Cellophane noodles
Channa flour

USEFUL GRAINS, GRAINS, NUTS, SEEDS, BEANS LEGUMES
Chestnut
Chia
Chickpea
Chickpea flour
Clear noodles
Coconut flour
Coffee alternatives
Colocasia esculenta (taro)
Corn bread organic Ø GMO
Corn meal organic Ø GMO
Corn organic Ø GMO
Corn tortillas organic Ø GMO
Crêpes buckwheat Ø wheat

USEFUL GRAINS, GRAINS, NUTS, SEEDS, BEANS LEGUMES
Dal
Dasheen araimo (taro)
Dinkel
Einkorn (spelt)
Emmer (farro)
English peas
Farro soak
Fava soak and peel
Flageolets soak
Forbidden rice~caution ↑ arsenic
GABA rice~caution ↑ arsenic
Gabi taro
Garbanzo beans chickpeas

USEFUL GRAINS, GRAINS, NUTS, SEEDS, BEANS LEGUMES
Garbanzo flour
Grain whole except wheat
Gram flour
Great northern bean
Green brown lentils
Grits organic Ø GMO
Groats
Hazelnut
Hempseed
Injera
Kamut
Kidney beans
Lentils

USEFUL GRAINS, GRAINS, NUTS, SEEDS, BEANS LEGUMES
Lima bean
Long bean threads
Lung kow noodles
Long kow vermicelli
Lotus root
Manihot esculenta, cassava
Marrow beans
Masa maiz
Mochi brown rice caution ↑ arsenic
Mung bean noodles
Mung beans
Navy beans
Northern beans

USEFUL GRAINS, GRAINS, NUTS, SEEDS, BEANS LEGUMES
Oats
Orange lentils
Pasta spelt, kamut, rye Ø wheat
Pasta whole grain Ø wheat
Peas
Pinto bean
Polenta organic Ø GMO
Popcorn organic caution aflatoxin, Ø salt
Potatoes sweet
Potatoes sweet jewel
Potatoes sweet Okinawan
Quinoa
Red bean soak for 3 days

USEFUL GRAINS, GRAINS, NUTS, SEEDS, BEANS LEGUMES
Red lentils
Red rice (not yeast) caution ↑ arsenic
Rice crackers Ø yeast wheat caution ↑ arsenic
Rye
Rye bread Ø yeast wheat
Rye crackers Ø yeast wheat
Rye crisps Ø yeast wheat
Sago root tapioca
Soba noodles
Spelt
Spelt bread Ø yeast
Spelt crackers Ø yeast flaxseed
Spelt pasta

USEFUL GRAINS, GRAINS, NUTS, SEEDS, BEANS LEGUMES
Spelt stuffing Ø yeast wheat
Stuffing Ø wheat
Sunchoke flour
Tapioca
Taro root
Teff
Ube
Vermicelli clear
White beans
White yam
Whole grains organic Ø wheat
Wild rice
Yam

USEFUL GRAINS, GRAINS, NUTS, SEEDS, BEANS LEGUMES
Yuca

👍 especially usef

13. USEFUL CHEMICALS

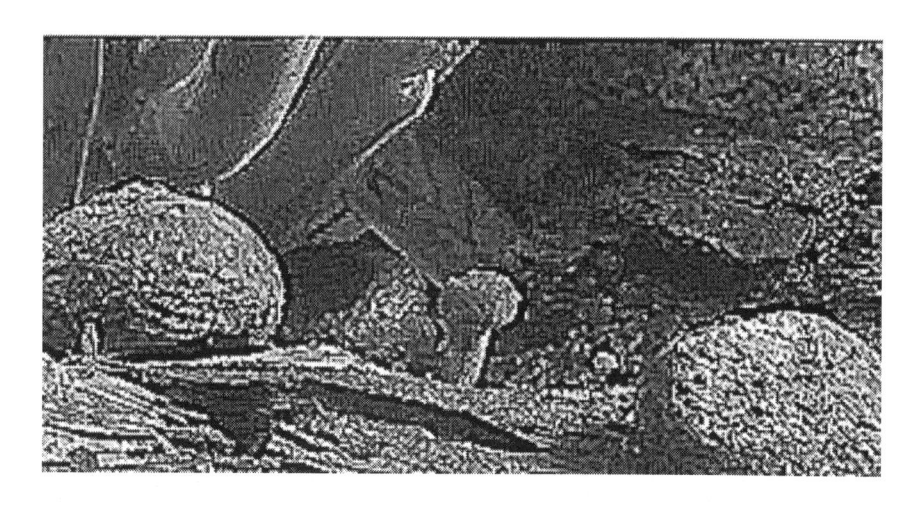

USEFUL CHEMICALS
ACE
ACEi caution elderly
Albumin
Alkalinity
Almond milk ice cream Ø carrageenan
Almond oil
Almond yogurt Ø carrageenan
Amino acids ↑ kidney functioning
Anti inflammatory foods
Antibiotics when needed
Aojiru
ARB angiotensin receptor site blockers
Arginex
Arrowroot
Ascorbic acid

USEFUL CHEMICALS
Avocado oil
Barley powder
Beneficial PKD
Bentonite clay
Biodynamic
Biomagnet pairs
Biotin
Blue zone
Bon ami
Borax
Boron
Brisdelle (paroxetine)
Broccoli DIMs
Burdock oil
Calcium citrate
Calcium in vegan foods
Cannabidiol
Charlotte's web
Chia oil
Chia oil capsules
Cobalamin
Coconut aminos
Coconut butter
Coenzyme Q10

USEFUL CHEMICALS
Colgate wisp miniToothbrush
CoQ10
Curcumin
Daiya
Date sugar
DIMs (broccoli sprouts)
Dr. Collins Restore toothpaste
Ecoplast
Elderberry syrup
Emu oil
Erythropoietin
Floradix
Fluoride carrageenan free toothpaste
Food restricted
Fuzzy toothbrush
Garlic oil
Gelatin
Ghassoul
Grape seed extract
H2 blockers
Hempseed oil
Hempseed oil capsules
Inositol
Iron foods

USEFUL CHEMICALS
Iron innate iron response when prescribed
Klettenwurzel haar oil
Lanreotide
Lemon egg
Leucine
Liver useful
Low fat
Lutein
Lycopene
Magnesium citrate (if OK)
Magnesium oil (if OK)
Magnet pairs
Menaquinone Ø soy
Meso-zeaxanthin
Miraculin
Moroccan Red Clay
Naringenin
Nattokinase Ø Soy
Nettle extract non alcoholic
Nexium
Niacin
Nicotinamide
NMN Nicotinamide Mononucleotide
O3 Pure Ozone laundry

USEFUL CHEMICALS
Octreotide
Oil almond
Oil hemp seed (raw)
Olive oil
Pantoprazole
Paroxetine
Pasireotide (wait)
Pepcid
Potassium citrate
Prebiotics
Prilosec
Proteinuria ↓
Proton pump inhibitors
Protonix
Pumpkin seed oil
Pyridoxine
Rhassoul clay
Riboflavin
Rutin
Samsca (caution liver)
Sandostatin LAR
Shohl's
Sodium Citrate
Solé
Test alkalinity

USEFUL CHEMICALS
Test blood pressure
Test proteinuria
Thiamine
Tight blood pressure control
Tolvaptan caution liver
Vasopressin suppression
Venlafaxine (Effexor)
Vitamin B1
Vitamin B12
Vitamin B2
Vitamin B6
Vitamin B7
Vitamin C
Vitamin D (if prescribed)
Vitamin E
Washing soda
Yoga
Zantac
Zeaxanthin
Zegerid

14. USEFUL VEGETABLES

USEFUL VEGETABLES
Acorn squash
Agaricus bisporus (crimini)
Anti-inflammatory foods
Artichoke
Artichokes globe
Artichokes Jerusalem
Artichokes sunchokes
Artocarpus altilis (breadfruit)
Arugula
Asparagus
Baby spring greens
Bamboo shoots
Bean sprouts
Beans green beans
Beans string beans
Beet greens ↑ oxalates
Beetroot
Bitter melon
Bok choy
Brassica
Breadfruit

USEFUL VEGETABLES

Breadnut
Broccoli
Broccoli rabe
Broccoli sprouts
Brussels sprouts
Buckwheat sprouts
Buddha's hand
Burdock root
Button mushrooms
Cabbage
Cabbage Chinese
Cabbage red
Cabbage savoy
Cantharellus cibarius (chanterelle)
Cardoons
Carrots
Cauliflower
Celeriac
Cèpes mushrooms
Chanterelle mushrooms
Chard
Chayote squash
Chicory
Chinese cabbage
Chinese peas

USEFUL VEGETABLES

Collard greens
Colocasia esculenta (taro)
Corn (non GMO)
Corn salad nüssli mache
Creasy greens
Crimini
Crookneck squash
Cruciferous vegetables
Cucumber Ø peel
Daikon radish
Dasheen araimo (taro)
Deadnettle
Delicata squash
Drumstick plant
Dryland cress
Eddoes
Edible flowers
Endive chicory
English peas
Escarole
Gabi
Girasole (sunchoke)
Globe artichoke
Gobi
Green beans

USEFUL VEGETABLES
Greens collard
Greens kale
Greens leafy
Greens mustard
Greens purslane
Haricots verts
Hearts of palm
Helianthus tuberosus (sunchoke)
Jerusalem artichokes
Jicama
Kabocha squash
Kale
Kohlrabi
Komatsuna
Lamb's lettuce
Land cress
Leafy greens
Leeks
Lettuce butter
Lettuce curly leaf
Lettuce mache lamb's lettuce
Lettuce oak leaf
Lettuce romaine
Lotus root

USEFUL VEGETABLES

Mache

Malungai

Malunggay leaves

Manihot esculenta

Manihot esculenta (yuca)

Manioc, cassava, yuca

Mixed wild greens

Mizuna

Morchella

Morels

Moringa oleifera

Mung bean sprouts

Murungai leaves

Mushrooms edible

Mustard greens

Napa

Nasturtiums

Nettle ↓ uric acid

Nüssli

Okinawan sweet potato

Okra

Olive caution salt

Onion

Opo

Oyster plants

USEFUL VEGETABLES
Pak choi
Parsnip
Pea
Porcini mushrooms
Portobello mushrooms
Potato sweet
Potatoes sweet jewel
Potatoes sweet Okinawan
Pumpkin
Purslane
Radish
Ramps
Rapini
Raw produce wash
Red cabbage
Red deadnettle
Red kuri pumpkin
Red onion
Rhizomes
Romaine lettuce
Rutabaga
Sago root, sago tapioca
Salsify, oyster plant, goatsbeard
Savoy cabbage
Scallions

USEFUL VEGETABLES
Shallots
Snap peas
Snow peas
Spring onions
Sprouts broccoli
Sprouts chickpea
Sprouts corn Ø GMO
Sprouts mung beans
Sprouts pea
Sprouts radish
Squash
Stinging nettle
String beans
Succotash
Sunchoke
Swedes
Sweet potato
Swiss chard
Tannia root
Tapioca
Taro root
Truffle
Turban squash
Turnip
Turnip greens

USEFUL VEGETABLES
Ube
Vegan cream cheese Ø soy
Vegetable korma
Vegetable pakora
Water chestnuts
Watercress
Wax beans
Welch onion, scallions
White asparagus
White carrots
White mushrooms
White radish
White yam
Wild onion ramps
Winter squash
Yam
Yellow onion
Yellow squash
Yuca
Zucchini Ø GMO

15. USEFUL FRUITS

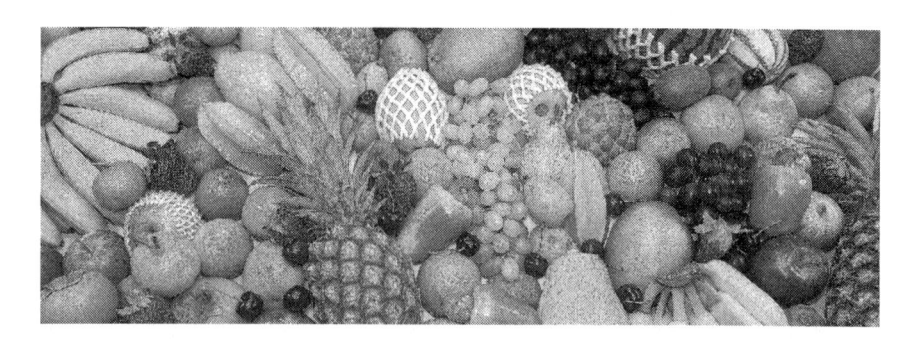

USEFUL FRUITS
Acerola
All fruit spread
Apple
Apple banana
Apple sauce
Apples sweet
Apricot
Avocado
Banana
Bartlett pear
Berries
Bing cherries
Black currants
Black raspberry
Blackberry
Boysenberry
Buddha's hand

USEFUL FRUITS
Calamansi
Cantaloupe local
Casaba melon local
Cherimoya
Cherry
Cherry Montmorency
Cherry sour
Chico
Citrus fruits
Clementine
Coconut
Currants
Custard apple
Dates
Donut peaches
Dragon fruit
Dried fruit
Durian
Figs fresh
Fruit
Fruit dried
Fuji apples
Gac
Gala apples
Golden delicious apple

USEFUL FRUITS
Golden raspberry
Gooseberry
Grape
Grapefruit
Gravenstein apple
Guava
Honeydew melon
Jackfruit
Kiwi
Kumquat
Langka
Lemon
Lemon Meyer
Lilikoi
Lime
Loquat
Mandarins
Mango
Mangosteen
Manilkara zapota sapodilla (chico)
Melon smooth skinned
Meyer lemon
Miracle berry
Montmorency cherry
Mulberry
Naval orange

USEFUL FRUITS
Nectarine
Orange
Papaya
Passion fruit
Paw paw
Peach
Pear
Persimmon
Pineapple
Pink apples
Pitihaya
Plantain
Pomelo
Queen Anne cherries
Quince
Rainier cherry
Raisin
Raspberry
Red banana
Red currants
Sapodilla (chico)
Sapote
Saturn peach
Smooth melon
Sour cherry
Tangelo

USEFUL FRUITS
Tsamma
Ugli
Watermelon
White nectarines
White peaches
Yellow currants
Zapota (chico)

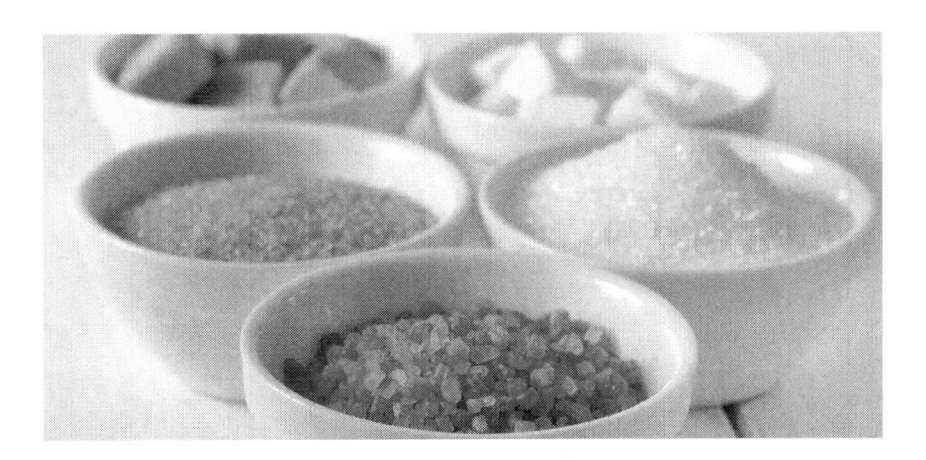

16. USEFUL SWEETENERS

ENJOY SWEETENERS
Apple sauce
Apple concentrate
Banana
Cinnamon
Date sugar
Dates
Miraculin
Miracle berries
Raisins
Tupelo honey

17. BETTER PROTEIN CHOICES

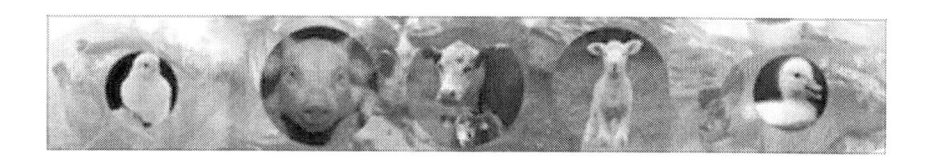

It is best to avoid animal proteins. If you are unable to do this, limit animal proteins to 3 ounces/day, twice a week. If dairy or cheese is eaten, these are limited to one ounce, or the size of one dice. Soft white cheese is preferable to dry yellow cheese

Better Protein Choices	Poorer Protein Choices
Daiya Vegan Cheese	Blue cheese
Miyoko Vegan Cheese	Mozzarella cheese
Follow my heart Vegan	Blue veined cheese
Almond Cheese	Cottage cheese
Almond Cheese	Ementhaler cheese
Almond Cheese	Feta cheese
Almond Cheese	Goat cheese
Almond Cheese	Paneer cheese
Almond Cheese	Quark cheese
Coconut milk	Cow or goat milk
Almond cheese	Sheep cheese
Coconut cheese	Soft white cheese

Better Protein Choices	Poorer Protein Choices
Almond milk lemon juice	Cultured buttermilk
Almond yogurt plain	Animal milk yogurt
Plain yogurt	Animal milk yogurt
Roquefort	Parmesan cheese
Swiss cheese	Romano cheese
Sheep cheese	Reggiani
Soft white cheese	Dry hard cheese
Blue cheese	Asiago cheese
Blue veined cheese	Dry cheese
Cottage cheese	Cheddar cheese
Dairy cultured	Best avoid animal dairy
Ementhaler	Orange yellow cheese
Feta salt & fat free	Mimolette cheese
Goat cheese	Mizithra cheese
Goat milk	Cow milk
Plant milk	Animal milk

Better Protein Choices	Poorer Protein Choices
Paneer plant cheese	Cheddar cheese
Quark cheese	Kefalotyn
Lamb	Beef
Veggie burger	Hamburger
Halibut Pacific	Salmon
Egg yolk poached	Scrambled egg
Wild turkey	Commercial poultry
Wild pheasant	Commercial pheasant

18. HELPS WITH PKD

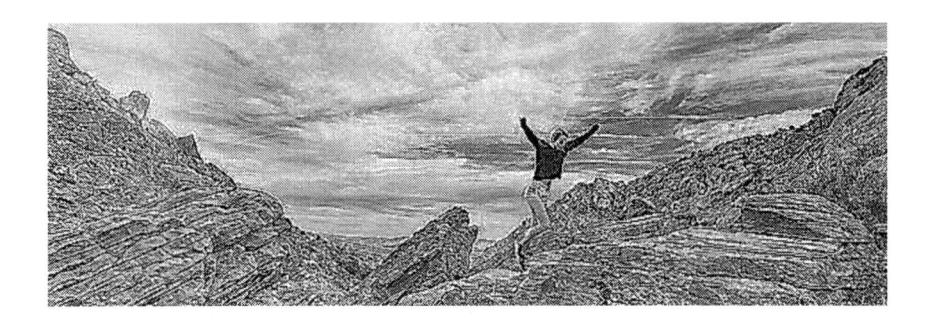

CLAY: Bentonite, pascalite, white, rhassoul, clay baths, hair masques.

SAUNAS: Dry saunas, steam saunas, useful for ↓ body toxins.

MASSAGE: Gentle relaxing massage.

REST: Restore yourself through rest, gentle stretches, sleep, restorative yoga

19. PKD CLINICAL TRIALS

ClinicalTrials.gov
A service of the U.S. National Institutes of Health

Clinical Trials for PKD
ACEi Angiotensin converting enzyme inhibitor ARB
Alkalinity
Colchicine (wait for trial completion)
DIMs
Leucine
Naringenin citrus fruits melons
Octreotide + Tolvaptan
Pioglitazone (wait)
Pix5568 - Plexikkon
Reversin (wait)

Clinical Trials for PKD
Roscovitine (wait)
Stem cells (wait)
Tight blood pressure
Tolvaptan Samsca (caution with liver disease) 👍
Triptolide (wait)
Vitamin B3 Niacin (wait)
Water
Pain Trial for PKD 👍

20. AVOID ITEMS WITH PKD

To follow are a list of items to be avoided with PKD. We know that these are to be avoided as this list of items does seem to increase symptoms from PKD. We with PKD have spent our time testing each item daily by measuring our abdominal girth at the same time at the same point and we have each made note if we experienced any pain or girth changes or kidney changes. To read further about these items try:
    AlkalineDiet.com/avoid.html or PKDiet.com/foods.php
    PKDiet.com/foods_herbs.pnp or PKDiet.com/foods_otc.php

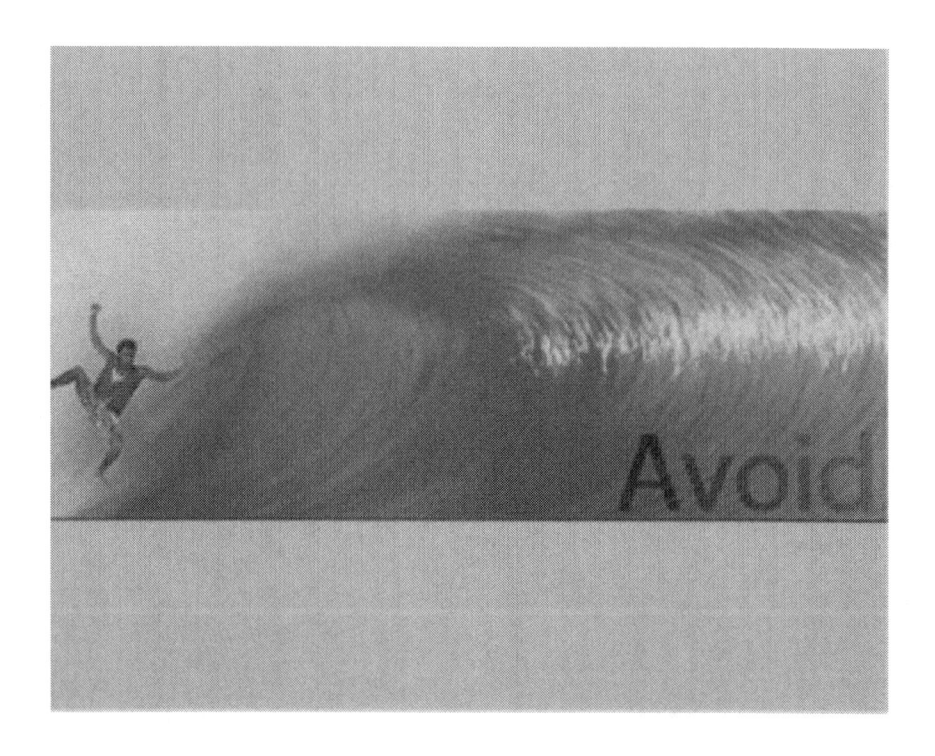

AVOID WITH PKD

3-benzylidene-camphor

4-Methylbenzylidene sunscn

Acacia fiber

Açai

Açai herb

Açai smoothie

Acesulfame potassium

Acetaminophen

Acetylsalicylic acid

Achyrocline

Ackee

Acrylamide

ADA azodicarbonamide

Advil

Aesculus hippocastanum

Afinitor® (everolimus)

Aflatoxin

African autumn tea

African nectar tea

Agave

Agave cactus

Aging (NMN)

Ahi tuna

Air fresheners phthalates

Alaskan king crab

Albacore tuna

AVOID WITH PKD

Alcohol

Alcohol aerosol

Alcohol methanol

Aldomet

Ale grain

Aleve

Alfalfa sprouts

Algae

Alkylphenols

All purpose flour

Allspice

Almond ice cream with carrageenan

Almond with aflatoxin

Aloe vera Ø eat

Aluminum

Amalgam

Amino Acid L-arginine

Amino Acid L-canavanine

Amino Acid L-carnitine

Amiodarone

Ammonia

Anabolic steroids

Anchovies

Andouille sausage

Angelica dong quai

AVOID WITH PKD
Animal proteins
Annatto
Anti-inflammatory medication
Antifreeze
Apple hard cider
Apple pie
Apple strudel
Arabitol
Aragonite all natural clay toothpaste
Arginine
Aristolochia
Aronia melanocarpa chokeberry
Arsenic
Artificial sweetener
Ashwagandha
Asiago cheese
Aspartame (Nutrasweet)
Aspergillus
Aspirin
Assugrin
Atrazine run off in water supply
Atrazine weed killer
Atta bulgur
Atta durum

AVOID WITH PKD

Atta flour

Aubergine

Auricularia polytricha (black fungus)

Autumn crocus only if needed by prescription

Aveeno nat mineral block face stick

Azodicarbonamide ADA

Bacon

Baguette wheat & yeast

Baked potato

Baking soda taken regularly

Bamboo rice

Bambu®

Banana split

Basil

Bathroom spray

BBQ

Bearberry

Beef

Beef hot dog

Beef pie

Beer grain

Beet sugar GMO

Bell peppers

Berberine

Bergamot

AVOID WITH PKD
BGH bovine growth hormone
BHA Butylated Hydroxyanisole
Bhatoora
Bhatura
BHT Butylated hydroxytoluene
Bihon
Bilberry whole fruit
Bio-oil®
Birth control pills
Bisacodyl
Bisphenol A (BPA) plastic
Black cohosh
Black fungus
Black pepper caution aflatoxin
Black seed & oil
Black tea
Blackstrap molasses
Bleach
Bleach cleanser
Bleached flour
Blood dishes
Blue-green algae
Blueberry whole fruit
Bluefish ↑ mercury
Bologna
Bonito

AVOID WITH PKD
Borage
Botanique toothpaste
Bottled juices methanol
Bovine growth hormone
BPA Bisphenol A plastic
Braggs apple cider vinegar
Braggs liquid aminos
Brahmi
Brake fluid
Bratwurst
Brazil nuts caution aflatoxin
Bread flour
Bread pudding
Brinjal eggplant
Brown rice syrup ↑ arsenic
Brown sugar
Brownies
Buchu
Buckthorn
Bud-nip
Bulgur wheat
Bundt cake
Bust enhancing herbs
Butter
ButylatedHydroxyanisole BHA
Cacao

AVOID WITH PKD
Cadmium
Caffeinated drink
Caffeine
Cake
Cake flour
Calendula
Callilepis laureola (Impila)
Calzone
cAMP
Canadian bacon
Canavanine
Candy
Cane juice crystals
Cane juices
Cane sugar
Canned drinks
Canned goods ↑ methanol
Canned juice esp ↑ methanol
Canned meat/soups ↑ methanol BHT
Canned vegetables ↑ methanol
Cannelloni
Cannoli
Canola oil
Cantaloupe fungus transported
Cape gooseberry (poha)
Capers

AVOID WITH PKD

Cappuccino

Capsicum annuum

Carambola

Caramels

Carbamazepine (tegretol)

Carbon tetrachloride

Carbonated sodas

Carnitine

Carrageenan

Carrot cake

Carrots dipped in bleach

Cascara sagrada

Casein

Cashew caution aflatoxin

Catchweed

Catfish

Cats claw

Catsfoot

Cayenne pepper

Celandine

Celery

Celery juice

Celery leaf

Cereal caution aflatoxin

Chaga mushroom/tea/powder

Chaparral

AVOID WITH PKD
Chaparral tea
Chapati
Charred meats
Chaste-tree berry
Cheddar cheese
Cheerios
Cheese
Cheese orange
Cheese parmesan
Cheese puffs
Cheeseburger
Cheesecake
Cheesesteaks
Chemicals ↑ cough
Chervil
Chicken (dipped in chlorine bath)
Chicken nuggets
Chicken sausage
Chili
Chinese gun powder tea
Chinese herbs
Chips salted
Chitosan
Chlorella
Chloride
Chlorine comet

AVOID WITH PKD
Chlorpropham
Chlorpyrifos
Chocolate
Chocolate cake
Chocolate chip cookies
Chocolate cookies
Chocolate cupcakes
Chocolate dipped strawberries
Chocolate éclairs
Chocolate flourless cake
Chocolate milk
Chocolate mousse
Chocolate truffles
Chokeberry whole fruit
Chondroitin
Chorizo
Chowder with dairy
Chrysanthemum tea
Cigarettes cigars chewing tobacco
Cimetidine
Clam juice
Clams
Cleanser with bleach
ClearLax
Cleaver
Clenz-Lyte

AVOID WUTH PKD
Clotted cream
Cloud ear fungus
Clover
Clover honey
Clover sprouts
Cloves
Co-Lav
Coca cola
Cocktails
Cocoa caution aflatoxin
Coconut ice cream with carrageenan
Coconut oil
Coconut sugar
Cod
Cod liver oil
Coffee ↑ estradiol 70%
Coffee beans
Cohosh
Cola drinks
Cola nut
Colase®
Colax
Colchicine only if needed by prescription
Colchicum only if needed by prescription
Coleus
Colgate toothpaste

AVOID WITH PKD
Colovage
Coltsfoot
Colyte
Comet cleanser
Comfrey ↓ liver functioning
Commercial poultry dipped in bleach
Concentrated sugar
Constipation
Cookies
Coral calcium
Coral white toothpaste
Cordarone (Amiodarone)
Cordyceps (fungi)
Corn bread GMO caution aflatoxin
Corn dumplings GMO caution aflatoxin
Corn GMO caution aflatoxin
Corn starch noodles
Corn syrup
Corned beef
Corydalis
Cosmetics phenoxyethanol
Cosmetics with cod liver oil
Cottonseed caution aflatoxin
Country mallow
Couscous
Crab

AVOID WITH PKD

Cracker meal
Cranberry pills
Cranberry whole fruit
Cream
Cream cheese
Cream of tartar
Cream puffs
Creamsicle
Creatine supplements
Créme fraiche
Crest toothpaste
Crisco
Croissant
Crustaceans
Cupcakes
Custard
Cyclamate
Cyclic AMP
Dairy
Dandelion greens
Danish
Daptacel vaccine (Phenoxyethanol)
Dark chocolate
Dashi
DCA Dichloroacetate in tap water

AVOID WITH PKD
DDE insecticide residue
DDT (dichlorodiphenyltrichloroethane)
Decaf coffee
Decaf cola
Decaf drinks
Decaf tea
DEHP PVC
Deli meat
Demerara sugar
Dessert sugar wheat
Detergents
Devil's claw
Dextrose
Dichloroacetate DCA
Dichlorodiphenyldichloroethane DDD
Dieldrin insecticide
Diethyl phthalate
Diethylstilbestrol
Diflucan
Dill
Dill pickles
Dong quai
Donuts
Doxidan

AVOID WITH PKD
DPA Diphenylamine
DPT Diphenylthiazole
Dr. Pepper
Dreamsicle
Dried fruit
Dried plum
Dried prune
Dried strawberry
Dry cleaned clothing/chemicals
Dryer sheets
Dubliner cheese
Duck
Dulcolax
Durum
E-Z-Em Fortrans
Echinacea
Éclair
Ecstasy
Edamame
Eel
Egg
Egg raw
Egg scrambled
Egg white
Eggnog
Eggplant

AVOID WITH PKD

Elderberry whole fruit
Enchiladas
Endocrine disruptors
Endosulfan (insecticide)
Energy drinks
Enriched flour
Ensure
Ephedra Sinica ↑BP
Equal
Erythritol
Erythrosine FD C Red 3
Escargot
Espresso
Essiac
Estrace
Estrogen
Estrogen BCP/pill/patch
Estrogen disruptors
Estrogenic shampoo
Ethanol
Ethylene glycol
Eugenol (oil cloves)
Everolimus
Excedrin
Fabric softener
Face cream

AVOID WITH PKD
Famotidine
Farina
Fats
Fennel
Fennel seed tea
Fenugreek
Fermented products, fish paste
Fettuccine wheat
Figs dried caution aflatoxin
Filet mignon
Fish
Fish anchovies
Fish cod liver oil
Fish mackerel
Fish oil
Fish salmon farmed esp. harmful
Fish sardines
Fish trout
Fish tuna
Flagyl
Flax seed
Flax seed crackers
Flax seed oil capsules
Flounder
Flour tortillas wheat
Fluconazole

AVOID WITH PKD
Fluoride
Fo ti
Fontina cheese
Foods heated in plastic
Formaldehyde
Forskolin
Fragrance
Fragrance BHT
Fragrance Diethyl phthalate
Fragrance Limonene
Fragrance Octinoxate
Fragrance Oxybenzone
Franks
French fries
Fried egg
Fried egg white
Fried foods
Fried vegetables
Fructose
Fruit caution
Fruit dried caution aflatoxin
Fudge
Fudgsicle
Galactitol
Galium aparine (cleavers)
Ganoderma lucidum

AVOID WITH PKD
Garcinia cambogia
GaviLax
Gavilyte
Gelato
Genistein (soy)
Gentamicin
Germander
Germanium
Ghee
Ginger ↑BP
Ginger ale
Ginkgo biloba
Ginseng ↑BP
Glechoma hederacea
Glucosamine
Glycolax
Glycols polyethylene → polyester
GlycoPrep
Glyphosate
GMO genetically modified
GMO seeds
Gnocchi
Go-Evac
Goji berries
Golden yukon potato
Goldenseal

AVOID WITH PKD
GoLYTELY®
Goosegrass
Gotu kola
Graham crackers
Graham flour
Grain beverage bambu
Grain beverage faux joe
Grain beverage postum
Grain beverage soyfee
Grain beverage yannoh
Grape seed oil
Grapefruit caution
Grapefruit juice caution
Graviola soursop
Green leaf tea
Green rice
Ground Ivy
Ground meat poultry fish
Groundnuts caution aflatoxin
Groundsel
Grouper ↑ mercury
Guar bean
Guar gum
Guarana
Hair dye chemicals
Hair gel

AVOID WITH PKD
HalfLytely
Ham
Ham hocks
Hamburger turkey burger fish burger
Hard cheese
Hard cider
Harmful herb tea acai mango zinger
Harmful herb tea African Autumn
Harmful herb tea African Nectar
Harmful herb tea Bengal spice
Harmful herb tea black cherry berry
Harmful herb tea caffeine free
Harmful herb tea chaparral
Harmful herb tea chocolate mint truffle
Harmful herb tea chrysanthemum
Harmful herb tea cinnamon apple spice
Harmful herb tea country peach
Harmful herb tea cranberry apple zinger
Harmful herb tea Essiac
Harmful herb tea fast lane black
Harmful herb tea fennel seed tea
Harmful herb tea guarana
Harmful herb tea honeybush
Harmful herb tea honeyVanillaChamomile
Harmful herb tea jammin lemon ginger

AVOID WITH PKD
Harmful herb tea lemon herbal love lemon
Harmful herb tea lemon verbena
Harmful herb tea lemon zinger
Harmful herb tea licorice root
Harmful herb tea maca
Harmful herb tea mama bear's cold care
Harmful herb tea mandarin orange spice
Harmful herb tea metabo balance
Harmful herb tea morning thunder
Harmful herb tea raspberry zinger
Harmful herb tea red clover
Harmful herb tea red tea
Harmful herb tea red zinger
Harmful herb tea redbush
Harmful herb tea roastaroma
Harmful herb tea rooibos
Harmful herb tea rooibos chai
Harmful herb tea sarsaparilla
Harmful herb tea sassafras
Harmful herb tea sleepytime
Harmful herb tea sleepytime kids grape
Harmful herb tea sleepytime peach
Harmful herb tea sleepytime vanilla
Harmful herb tea sweet apple chamomile
Harmful herb tea tangerine orange zinger
Harmful herb tea tension tamer

AVOID WITH PKD
Harmful herb tea true blueberry
Harmful herb tea wild berry zinger
Harmful herb tea yerba mate
Harmful tea black
Harmful tea caffeine
Harmful tea Chinese gunpowder
Harmful tea decaffeinated
Harmful tea Earl Gray tea
Harmful tea green
Harmful white tea
Harpagophytum
Hash browns
Hawthorne ↑BP
Heating food in microwave
Helianthus annuus L
Heptachlor (insecticide)
Herbicides
Herring
Hershey bars
HFCS High fructose corn syrup
Hoagies
Homocysteine
Hops
Hormone
Horse chestnut
Horseradish

AVOID WITH PKD
Horsetail
Hot chocolate
Hot dogs, rindswurst
Hot fudge sundae
Hot tamales with lard
Hot toddy
HRT
Huckleberry whole fruit
Hydrogenated starch hydrolysate HSH
Hydrolyzed wheat protein
Ibuprofen
Ice cream
Ice cream drumstick
Iceberg lettuce
Imitrex
Impila root
Inflammatory foods
Isomalt
Italian sausage
Ivy
Jaggery
Jalapeño pepper
Jason Oral comfort toothpaste
Jason PowerSmile toothpaste
Jin Bu Huan
Juice bottled/canned (BPA)

AVOID WITH PKD
Juniper
Just like sugar
Kava-kava
Keishi-bukuryo
Ketoconazole
Kidney avoid
Kiss my face toothpaste
Kola nut
Kombu (dashi, bonito flakes)
Kombucha
Krameria triandra (rhatany root)
Kudzu
Kwao krua kao
L-arginine
L-canavanine
L-canitine
L'oreal HiP High Intensity Pigments
L'amour encage
Lactitol
Lady fingers
Langoustines
Lanzones
Lard
Lasagna
Lassi
Latté

AVOID WITH PKD
Laundry powder
Lavender
Lax Lyte
Lax-a-Day
Laxatives
Lead
Lecithin (soy)
Lectin
Lei gong teng (Wait)
Lemon verbena
Lesys (Maltitol, maltisweet, sweetPearl)
Lettuce exclude iceberg
Licorice ↑BP
Licorice drinks
Limonene → formaldehyde
Lindane (insecticide)
Lingzhi
Link sausage
Linseed
Linseed oil
Lithium
Liver
Liverwurst
Lobelia
Lobster

AVOID WITH PKD
Loco moco
Lollipop
Longan
Lovage
Luchi
Lupin
Lychee
Lysergic acid LSD
LytePrep
Ma Huang
Maca herb
Macaroni and cheese
Macaroni salad
Mace
Macela achyrocline satureoides
Mackerel ↑ mercury
Macrogol
Magnolia officinalis
Mai tai
Maize caution aflatoxin
Malasadas
Malt liquor
Maltisweet (Maltitol Lesys SweetPearl)
Maltitol
Mangosteen juice bottled
Manicotti

AVOID WITH PKD
Mannitol
Maple syrup
Maraschino cherries
Margarine
Marlin ↑ mercury
Masala dosa wheat & potato
Mate
Matzo
Matzo wheat
Meat red
Meatballs
Meatloaf
Mederma scar cream
Melaleuca
Melon transported develop fungus
Menaquinone
Mercury
Metalloestrogens
Methanol
Methanol alcoholic drinks
Methionine
Methoxychlor (insecticide)
Methyldopa
Methylisothiazolinone DNA damage
Methylparabens
Mexican chocolate

AVOID WITH PKD
Microwaved food
Microwaved popcorn
Migraine
Milk chocolate
Milk cow animal
Milk shakes animal milks
Millet
MiraLAX
Miso
Miso soup
Mistletoe
MIT Methylisothiazolinone
Mixed alcohol
Mixed alcohol methanol
MK7 with soy
Mochi white rice
Mochiko
Molasses
Monk fruit in the raw sweetener (contains dextrose)
Monster energy drink
Monterey jack cheese
Motherwort
Motrin
Mountain apple
Movicol

AVOID WITH PKD
MoviPrep
Mozzarella cheese
MSG (monosodium glutamate)
MSM (methylsulfonylmethane)
Mulberry whole fruit
Mullet
Multiple vitamins
Muscovado sugar
Mussels
Mycose
Myristica fragrans
N-nitrosomorpholine NNM
Naan
Nail chemicals polish removers
Naltrexone
Naproxen
Nattō from soy
Nattokinase
Natural dentist toothpaste
Natural tea tree toothpaste
Neatsfoot oil
Nectresse
Neem
Neem toothpaste
Neotame
Neutrogena body oil

AVOID WITH PKD
Neutrogena liquid facial cleanser
Niacin
Nicotinamide
Nigella sativa
Nightshade plants
Nitrites
Nitrosamine
Nizoral
NNM (N-nitrosomorpholine)
Non-dairy creamer
Non-stick teflon
Noni juice & fruit
Nonylphenol
Norbu
NSAID
NuLYTELY
Nutmeg
NutraSweet (aspartame)
Nutribiotic toothpaste
Nutritional yeast
OCL (laxative)
Octinoxate sunscreen
Oil canola
Oil coconut
Oil cottonseed
Oil grape seed
Oil lavender

AVOID WITH PKD
Oil palm
Oil safflower
Oil sesame
Oil sunflower
Oil tea tree oil (melaleuca)
Oilseeds caution aflatoxin
Oily fish
Olay daily facial cleaning cloth
Olives caution salt
Onion dip
Orange cheese
Orange roughy ↑ mercury
Organ meats
Organic chlorinated pesticides
Organophosphorus pesticides
Osha root
Ospemifene
Osphena™
Oven cleaners
Oxybenzone
Packaged vegetables chlorine bath
PAH Polycyclic arom hydrocarbon
Palm oil
Pancit
Panela
Papad

AVOID WITH PKD
Papadum
Paprika
Paraben
Paracetamol
Paratha
Parmesan cheese
Parmigiano Reggiano cheese
Parsley ↑ oxalates ↓BP
Pasta wheat
Pastrami
Paté foie gras
Patis
Pau d'arco
Peanut butter aflatoxin
Peanut butter cookies
Peanut butter cups
Peanut butter pretzels
Peanuts aflatoxin
Pecans aflatoxin
PEG
Peg Lyte
Pemmican
Pennyroyal
Pentachlorophenol
Pepcid
Pepino

AVOID WITH PKD
Pepperoni
Peppers
Perch
Perchlorate
Perfume
Perfuorinated chemicals PFC
PerioBrite toothpaste
Pesticides
Pheasant, commercial
Phenacetin
Phenol nonylphenol
Phenosulfothiazine red dye
Phenoxyethanol cosmetics
Phthalates plasticizers
Physalis peruviana (poha)
Phytates phytic acid
Phytoestrogens i.e. soy
Pickle juice
PIckled egg
Pickles
Pie made with lard, sugar, wheat
Piloncillo
Pimenta dioica
Pimento
Piña colada rum
Pink meats

AVOID WITH PKD

Pink slime
Pioglitazone (wait)
Pistachios caution aflatoxin
Pita, pita chips
Pizza wheat yeast tomatoes
Plastic all
Plastic wrap
Plexxicon PLX5568
Plum
Poha berry
Poke
Poke Root
Polychlorinated biphenyls
Polycyclic arom hydrocarbon PAH
Polyester
Polyethylene glycol
Polygonum Multiflorum (Fo-ti)
Pomegranate caution
Pomegranate juice
Poppadum
Poppyseed
Popsicle
Pork
Pork pie
Pork sausage
Portuguese sausage

AVOID WITH PKD
Potato
Potato chips
Potato flour
Potato salad
Poultry dipped bleach
Precut vegetables
Pregnancy
Premarin
Prempro
Prep lyte
Pretzels (salted wheat)
Prickly pear
Prime rib
Processed American cheese
Processed foods
Processed meats
Produce dipped in bleach
Progesterone (& creams)
Prosciutto
Provolone cheese
Prune
Prune butter
Prune juice
Pudding
PUFA Polyunsaturated fatty acids
Pumpkin pie & whipped cream

AVOID WITH PKD
Purelax
PureVia
Puri
PVC polyvinyl chloride
Pyridoxine
Quail
Quail eggs
Quarter pounder
Queen Anne's lace (wild carrot)
Raclette
Ractopamine
Ragu sauce
Ragwort
Rambutan
Ramen noodles
Rapadura
Rapamune
Rapamycin
Ravioli
Raw egg
Raw egg whites
Ready eat vegetables (bleach)
Red clover
Red clover tea honey
Red dye
Red meat

AVOID WITH PKD

Red pimento

Red velvet cake

Red yeast rice

Red/white potato

Redbush

Reggiano cheese

Reishi

Remifemin

Resveratrol

Reversin wait

Revlon ColorStay Bronzer for the Face

Rhatany

Rhubarb

Rice ice cream with carrageenan

Rice pudding

Rice syrup ↑ arsenic

Rice white ↑ arsenic

Rice wine ↑ arsenic

Rigatoni

Rindswurst

Roast beef pre-cooked

Rolls yeasted

Rolly toothpaste brush

Romano cheese

Rooibos

Root beer

AVOID WITH PKD
Roscovitine
Rosemary
Roti
Roundup®
Rum scotch gin methanol
Russet potato
S-adensylmethionine
Saccharin
Sage
Sake
Salami
Salmon farmed esp. harmful
Salt limit
Salt pork
Saltines
SAMe
Saran wrap
Sardines
Sarsaparilla
Sarsaparilla drinks
Sashimi
Sassafras
Sassafras drinks
Satureoides (Macela Achyrocline)
Sausage
Saw palmetto

AVOID WITH PKD

Scallops

Scampi

Scar bio oil

Scent fragrance

Scrambled egg white avitamin

Scrambled eggs

Sea Asparagus

Sea bass ↑ mercury

Seaweed ↑ mercury

Seitan

Seliciclib

Semolina

Senna

Sesame seed

Shampoo with formaldehyde

Shampoo with methylisothiazolinone MIT

Shampoo with methylparabens

Shampoo with parabens

Shampoo with phthalates

Shampoo with sodium lauryl sulfate

Shark ↑ mercury

Shell fish ↑ mercury

Shrimp ↑ mercury

Siberian ginseng

Silver amalgam

Sirolimus

AVOID WITH PKD
Skullcap
Sloppy Joe's
Smoothies with dairy sugar
Snakeroot
Soap powder
Soda pop
Sodium bicarbonate frequently
Sodium lauryl sulfate
Softlax
Sole (fish)
Solvent
Sorbitol (maltitol)
Sorrel dip in boiling water ↓ oxalates
Sour cream
Soursop
Soy
Soy beans
Soy flour
Soy lecithin
Soy milk
Soy sauce
Spaghetti meatballs/ meat sauce
Spaghetti sauce
Spaghetti wheat
SPAM
Spare ribs

AVOID WITH PKD
Spices caution aflatoxin
Spiker water resistant styling glue
Spinach
Spinach apple juice
Spirits
Spirulina
Splenda
Spray cleaners
Sprouts alfalfa
Sprouts clover
Sprouts soy
Squab
Squid
St. John's Wort
Star anise
Starfruit
Statins
Steak
Stephania tetrandra
Stevia
Stickyweed
Stout malt liquor
Strawberry
Strawberry drinks
Strawberry leaf
Stroganoff

AVOID WITH PKD
Stuffing with wheat
Styrofoam containers
Sucanat
Sucralose
Sucrose
Sugar
Sugar beets if GMO
Sugar cane
Sugar cane crystals
Sugar cane juice
Sugar cookies
Sugar twin
Sun chips
Sunett (asesulfame potassium, Ace-K)
Sunflower oil
Sunflower seeds
Sunscreen 4-Methylbenzylidene
Sunscreen benzophenone-3
Sushi
Swedish meatballs
Sweet clover
Sweet One
Sweet rolls yeast wheat
Sweet white rice
Sweet'N Low
SweetPearl (maltitol)

AVOID WITH PKD
Swordfish ↑ mercury
Syzygium aromaticum (clove)
Syzygium malaccense (Mt. apple)
T'u-san-chi
Table sugar
Taco
Tagamet
Tagatose sugar
Tagliatelle
Tahini
Tamales with fard tomatoes
Tamari
Tamarind
Tannia leaf (lobelia)
Tanqueray
Tansy
Tapioca drink coconut milk
Tarragon
Tea black
Tea caffeine
Tea decaffeinated
Tea green
Tea plant
Tea tree oil
Tea white
Teeth plastic fillings

AVOID WITH PKD
Teflon
Tegretol
Tempeh
Tequila
Tequila methanol
Teriyaki sauce
Tesevatinib (wait for trials)
Testosterone
Thymoquinone
Tilapia
Tilefish ↑ mercury
Tiramisu
TMAO Trimethylamine *N*-oxide
Tobacco
Tofu
Toll house cookies
Tom's toothpaste
Tomatillo
Tomato
Tomato juice
Tomatoes canned BHT methanol
Tortellini
Tortillas wheat
Tree nuts
Trehalose (mycose)
Tribulus Terrestris

AVOID WITH PKD

Triclosan in water supply

TriLyte

Triptolide (wait)

Triticum

Tropical mountain apple

Trout ↑ mercury

Truvia

Tuna ↑ mercury

Turbinado sugar

Turkey

Turkey bacon

Turkey sausage

Tylenol

Udon (buckwheat + wheat)

Uva Ursi

V8

Valerian

Vanilla extract

Veal

Veg juice bottle/canned BPA

Vegemite

Velveeta cheese

Vichyssoise

Vienna sausage

Vinegar

Vitamin B3

AVOID WITH PKD
Vitamin K2 with soy
Vitex agnus-castus
Vytorin
Walnuts caution aflatoxin
Water crackers
Wax jambu
Weedkiller
Wheat
Wheat bran
Wheat bread
Wheat germ
Wheat protein isolate
Wheatena
Whey
Whipped cream
White beet sugar
White cane sugar
White chocolate
White flour
White potato
White rice
White tea
Whiting
Wild boar
Wild carrot
Wild yam progesterone cream

AVOID WITH PKD
Willow bark
Windex
Window cleaners
Wine
Withania somnifera
Wolfberry
Wonton
Wood ear fungus
Woodruff
Worcestershire sauce
Wormseed
Wormwood
Xagave
Xanthan gum
Xenoestrogens
Xylitol
Xylitol spry toothpaste
Yeast
Yeasted baked goods
Yeasted breads
Yeasted breads
Yellow cheese
Yerba mate

AVOID WITH PKD
Yogurt with dairy
Yucca ornamental
Zucchini if GMO

21. AVOID ANIMAL PROTEINS

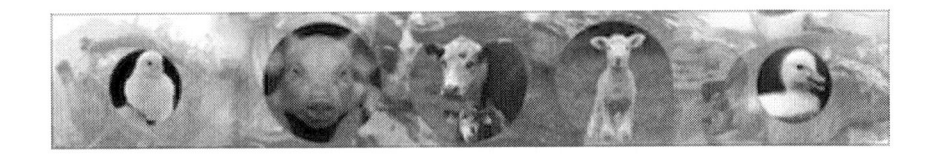

AVOID ANIMAL PROTEINS
Ahi tuna
Alaskan king crab
Albacore tuna
Anchovies
Andouille sausage
Animal proteins
Asiago cheese
Bacon
Banana split
BBQ
Beef
Beef hot dog
Beef/pork pie
Bihon
Blood dishes
Bluefish
Bologna
Bonito
Bratwurst

AVOID ANIMAL PROTEINS
Butter
Canadian bacon
Canned meat/soups ↑ methanol BHT
Catfish
Charred meats
Cheddar cheese
Cheese caution aflatoxin
Cheese orange
Cheese parmesan
Cheeseburger
Cheesecake
Cheeses
Cheesesteaks
Chicken (dipped in chlorine bath)
Chicken nuggets
Chicken sausage
Chocolate milk
Chocolate mousse
Chorizo
Chowder w/dairy
Clams
Clotted cream
Cod
Cod liver oil
Commercial poultry dipped in bleach
Corned beef

AVOID ANIMAL PROTEINS
Crab
Cream
Cream cheese
Creamsicle
Créme fraiche
Crustaceans
Custard
Dairy
Deli meat
Dreamsicle
Dubliner cheese
Duck
Éclair
Eel
Egg
Egg raw
Egg scrambled
Egg whites
Eggnog
Enchiladas
Escargot
Fermented fish paste
Filet mignon
Fish
Fish anchovies
Fish cod liver oil

AVOID ANIMAL PROTEINS
Fish oil
Fish salmon farmed esp. harmful
Fish sardines
Fish trout
Fish tuna
Flounder
Fontina cheese
Franks
Fried egg
Fried egg white
Fudge
Fudgsicle
Gelato
Ghee
Ground meat poultry fish
Grouper ↑ mercury
Ham
Ham hocks
Hamburger turkey burger, fish burger
Hard cheese
Herring
Hoagies
Hot chocolate
Hot dogs, rindswurst
Hot fudge sundae
Hot tamales w/lard

AVOID ANIMAL PROTEINS

Ice cream
Ice cream drumstick
Italian sausage
Kombu (dashi, bonito flakes)
Langoustines
Lard
Lasagna
Lassi
Latté
Link sausage
Liver
Liverwurst
Lobster
Loco moco
Macaroni and cheese
Mackerel ↑ mercury
Manicotti
Marlin ↑ mercury
Meat red
Meatballs
Meatloaf
Milk chocolate
Milk cow animal
Milk shakes animal milks
Monterey jack cheese
Mozzarella cheese
Mullet

AVOID ANIMAL PROTEINS
Mussels
Oily fish
Onion dip
Orange dry cheese
Orange roughy
Organ meats
Orange cheese
Orange roughy ↑ mercury
Organ meats
Pancit
Parmesan cheese
Parmigiano Reggiano cheese
Pastrami
Paté foie gras
Patis
Pemmican
Pepperoni
Perch
Pheasant, commercial
Pickled eggs
Pink meats
Pink slime
Poke
Pork
Pork pie
Pork sausage

AVOID ANIMAL PROTEINS

Portuguese sausage

Poultry dipped bleach

Prime rib

Processed American cheese

Processed meat

Prosciutto

Provolone cheese

Pudding

Quail

Quail eggs

Quarter pounder

Raclette

Ravioli

Raw egg

Raw egg whites

Red meat

Reggiano cheese

Rigatoni

Rindswurst

Roast beef pre-cooked

Romano cheese

Salami

Salmon farmed esp. harmful

Salt pork

Sardines

Sashimi

AVOID ANIMAL PROTEINS
Sausage
Scallops
Scampi
Scrambled egg white avitamin
Scrambled eggs
Sea bass ↑ mercury
Shark ↑ mercury
Shell fish ↑ mercury
Shrimp ↑ mercury
Sloppy Joe's
Smoothie dairy
Sole
Sour cream
Spaghetti meatballs/ meat sauce
SPAM
Spare ribs
Squab commercial
Squid
Steak
Sushi
Swedish meatballs
Swordfish ↑ mercury
Tacos
Tamale meat lard tomatoes
Tilapia
Tilefish

AVOID ANIMAL PROTEINS
Trout ↑ mercury
Tuna ↑ mercury
Turkey
Turkey bacon
Turkey sausage
Veal
Velveeta cheese
Vienna sausage
Whey
Whipped cream
Whiting
Wild boar
Wonton
Yellow hard dry cheese
Yogurt

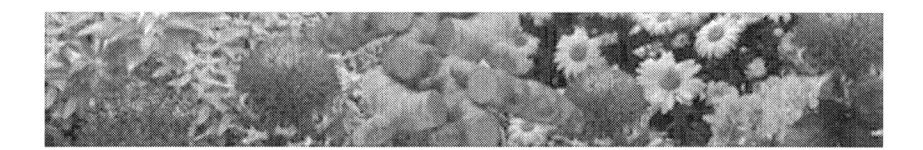

22. AVOID HERBS

AVOID HERBS
Acacia fiber
Açai herb
Achyrocline
Aesculus hippocastanum
Agave cactus
Alfalfa
Allspice
Aloe vera
Angelica dong quai
Annatto
Aristolochia
Aronia
Aronia melanocarpa chokeberry
Ashwagandha
Autumn crocus only if needed by prescription
Basil
Bearberry
Berberine
Bergamot
Black cohosh

AVOID HERBS
Black pepper caution aflatoxin
Black seed
Borage
Brahmi
Buchu
Buckthorn
Bust enhancing herbs
Cacao
Calendula
Callilepis laureola (Impila)
Cascara sagrada
Catchweed
Cats claw
Catsfoot
Cayenne pepper
Celandine
Celery leaf
Chaparral
Chaste-tree berry
Chervil
Chili
Chinese herbs
Chokeberry berries (juice is fine but berries too high in oxalates)
Chrysanthemum
Cleavers

AVOID HERBS
Clover
Cloves
Cohosh
Colchicum
Coleus
Coltsfoot
Comfrey ↓ liver functioning
Corydalis
Country mallow
Dandelion
Devil's claw
Dill
Dong quai
Echinacea
Ephedra sinica ↑BP
Fennel
Fenugreek
Flax
Fo ti
Forskolin
Galium aparine (cleavers)
Garcinia cambogia
Germander
Ginger ↑BP

AVOID HERBS
Ginkgo biloba
Ginseng ↑BP
Goji
Goldenseal
Goosegrass
Gotu kola
Ground ivy
Groundsel
Guarana
Harpagophytum
Hawthorn ↑BP
Hops
Horse chestnut
Horseradish
Horsetail
Impila root
Ivy
Jin Bu Huan
Juniper
Kava-kava
Keishi-bukuryo
Kola nut
Krameria triandra (rhatany root)
Kudzu
Kwao krua kao

AVOID HERBS

Lavender
Lei gong teng (Wait)
Lemon verbena
Licorice ↑BP
Linseed
Lobelia
Lovage
Lupin
Ma Huang
Maca herb
Mace
Macela achyrocline satureoides
Magnolia officinalis
Mate
Melaleuca
Mistletoe
Motherwort
Myristica fragrans
Neem
Nigella sativa
Nutmeg
Osha root
Paprika
Parsley ↑ oxalates ↓BP

AVOID HERBS
Pau d'arco
Pennyroyal
Pimenta dioica (allspice)
Poke Root
Polygonum multiflorum
Poppyseed
Queen Anne's lace (wild carrot)
Ragwort
Red clover
Redbush
Remifemin
Rhatany
Rooibos
Rosemary
Sage
Salt limit
Sarsaparilla
Sassafras
Satureoides
Saw palmetto
Senna
Siberian ginseng
Skullcap
Snakeroot

AVOID HERBS
Spices caution aflatoxin
St. John's Wort
Star anise
Stephania tetrandra
Stevia
Stickyweed
Strawberry leaf
Sweet clover
Syzygium aromaticum (clove)
T'u-san-chi
Tamarind
Tannia leaves
Tansy
Tarragon
Tea tree Oil
Tribulus Terrestris
Uva Ursi
Valerian
Vanilla extract
Vitex agnus-castus
Wild carrot
Willow bark
Withania somnifera
Woodruff

AVOID HERBS
Wormwood
Yerba mate
Yucca

24. AVOID GRAINS

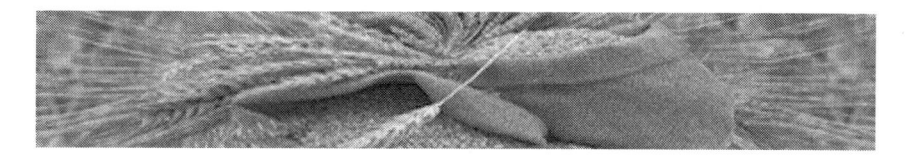

Soak to ↓ phytates; an increase in phytates can lead to a migraine.

AVOID GRAINS
All purpose flour
Almond dream
Almond ice cream carrageenan
Apple pie
Apple strudel
Atta bulgur
Atta durum
Atta flour
Baguette wheat
Baked potato
Bamboo rice
Bhatoora
Bhatura
Bihon
Bleached flour
Brazil nuts
Bread flour
Bread pudding
Brownies
Bulgur wheat

AVOID GRAINS

Bundt cake

Cake

Cake flour

Calzone

Cannelloni

Cannoli

Carrot cake

Cashew caution aflatoxin

Cereal caution aflatoxin

Cheerios

Cheese puffs

Cheesecake

Chips salted

Chocolate cake

Chocolate chip cookies

Chocolate cookies

Chocolate cupcakes

Chocolate éclairs

Chocolate flourless cake

Cookies

Corn bread GMO caution aflatoxin

Corn dumplings GMO caution aflatoxin

Corn GMO

Corn starch noodles

Couscous

Cracker meal

AVOID GRAINS

Cream puffs

Croissant

Cupcakes

Custard pie

Danish

Dessert wheat

Donuts

Durum

Éclair

Enchiladas

Enriched flour

Farina

Fettuccine wheat

Flaxseed

Flaxseed crackers

Flour tortillas wheat

Gnocchi

Graham crackers

Graham flour

Green rice

Groundnuts caution aflatoxin

Guar bean

Guar gum

Helianthus annuus L (sunflower seeds)

Hoagies

Hot tamales with lard

AVOID GRAINS
Lady fingers
Lasagna
Lecithin (soy)
Luchi
Macaroni and cheese
Macaroni salad
Maize caution aflatoxin
Malasadas
Manicotti
Masa maiz
Masala dosa with wheat & potato
Matza
Matzo wheat
Microwaved popcorn
Millet
Miso
Miso soup
Mochi white rice
Mochiko
Naan
Nattō soy
Nutritional yeast
Pancit
Papad
Papadum
Paratha

AVOID GRAINS
Paratha
Pasta wheat
Pasta whole grain wheat
Peanut butter
Peanut butter cookies
Peanut butter pretzels
Peanuts aflatoxin
Pecan aflatoxin
Pie made with lard, sugar, wheat
Pistachios caution aflatoxin
Pita, Pita chips
Pizza wheat yeast tomatoes
Poppadom
Poppyseed
Pork pie
Potato chips
Potato flour
Potato salad
Pretzels salted wheat
Pumpkin pie with whipped cream
Puri
Ramen noodles
Ravioli
Red velvet cake
Rice contains arsenic
Rice pudding

AVOID GRAINS
Rice white
Rigatoni
Rolls yeasted
Roti
Russet potato
Saltines
Seitan
Semolina wheat
Sesame seed
Sloppy Joe's
Soy
Soy beans
Soy flour
Soy lecithin
Spaghetti meatballs
Spaghetti wheat
Stroganoff
Stuffing with wheat
Sugar cookies
Sun chips
Sunflower seed
Sushi white rice
Sweet rolls yeast wheat
Sweet white rice
Tagliatelle
Tahini
Tamales with lard tomatoes

AVOID GRAINS
Tahari
Tempeh
Tiramisu
Tofu
Toll house cookies
Tortellini
Tortillas wheat
Tree nuts caution aflatoxin
Triticum (wheat)
Udon (buckwheat + wheat)
Vegemite
Walnuts aflatoxin
Water crackers
Wheat
Wheat bran
Wheat bread
Wheat germ
Wheat protein isolate
Wheat starch
Wheatena
White flour
White potato flour
White rice
Wonton
Xanthan gum
Yeast

AVOID GRAINS

Yeasted baked goods

Yeasted breads

25. AVOID DRINKS

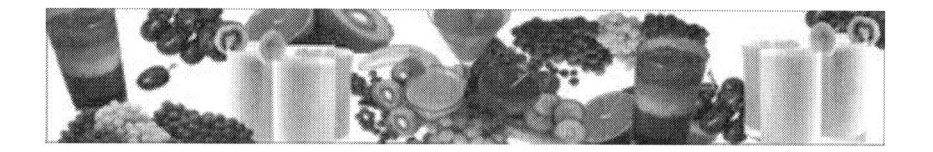

AVOID DRINKS
Açai smoothie
African autumn tea
African nectar tea
Alcohol
Alcohol methanol
Ale
Aloe Ø drink
Apple hard cider
Bambu
Beer
Black tea
Bottled juice
Caffeinated drink
Cane juice
Canned drinks
Canned juice esp ↑ methanol
Cappuccino
Carbonated sodas

AVOID DRINKS

Celery juice
Chaga mushroom tea
Chaparral tea
Chinese gunpowder tea
Chocolate drinks milk
Clam juice
Coca cola
Cocktails
Cocoa
Coffee ↑ estradiol 70%
Cola drinks
Cream
Dairy
Decaf coffee
Decaf cola
Decaf drink
Decaf tea
Dr. Pepper
Earl gray teas
Egg white raw
Eggnog
Energy drinks
Ensure

AVOID DRINKS
Espresso
Essiac
Ethanol
Ginger ale
Grain beverage bambu
Grain beverage faux joe
Grain beverage postum
Grain beverage soyKaffee
Grain beverage yannoh
Grapefruit juice caution
Green leaf tea
Hard cider
Harmful herb tea acai mango zinger
Harmful herb tea African Autumn
Harmful herb tea African Nectar
Harmful herb tea apple chamomile
Harmful herb tea Bengal spice
Harmful herb tea black cherry berry
Harmful herb tea caffeine free
Harmful herb tea chaparral
Harmful herb tea chocolate mint truffle
Harmful herb tea chrysanthemum
Harmful herb tea cinnamon apple spice

AVOID DRINKS
Harmful herb tea essiac
Harmful herb tea fast lane black
Harmful herb tea fennel seed tea
Harmful herb tea guarana
Harmful herb tea honeybush
Harmful herb tea honeyVanillaChamomile
Harmful herb tea jammin lemon ginger
Harmful herb tea lemon herbal love lemon
Harmful herb tea lemon verbena
Harmful herb tea lemon zinger
Harmful herb tea licorice root
Harmful herb tea maca
Harmful herb tea mama bear's cold care
Harmful herb tea mandarin orange spice
Harmful herb tea metabo balance
Harmful herb tea morning thunder
Harmful herb tea raspberry zinger
Harmful herb tea red clover
Harmful herb tea red tea
Harmful herb tea red zinger
Harmful herb tea redbush
Harmful herb tea roastaroma
Harmful herb tea rooibos chai
Harmful herb tea rooibos

AVOID DRINKS
Harmful herb tea sarsaparilla
Harmful herb tea sassafras
Harmful herb tea sleepytime
Harmful herb tea sleepytime kids grape
Harmful herb tea sleepytime peach
Harmful herb tea sleepytime vanilla
Harmful herb tea sweet apple chamomile
Harmful herb tea tangerine orange zinger
Harmful herb tea tension tamer
Harmful herb tea true blueberry
Harmful herb tea wild berry zinger
Harmful herb tea yerba mate
Harmful tea black
Harmful tea caffeine
Harmful tea Chinese gunpowder
Harmful tea decaffeinated
Harmful tea Earl Gray tea
Harmful tea green
Harmful tea white
Hot chocolate
Hot toddy
Juice bottled/canned BPA
Lassi
Latté

AVOID DRINKS
Licorice drinks
Mai tai
Malt liquor
Mangosteen juice bottled
Methanol
Methanol alcoholic drinks
Mexican hot chocolate
Milk cow animal
Milk shakes animal milks
Mixed alcohol methanol drinks
Monster energy drink
Noni juice
Pickle juice
Piña colada rum
Pomegranate juice
Prune juice
Raw egg
Raw egg whites
Red clover tea
Rice wine ↑ arsenic
Root beer
Rum scotch gin methanol
Saké
Sarsaparilla drinks
Sassafras drinks

AVOID DRINKS

Smoothies with dairy sugar
Soda pop
Soy milk
Spinach apple juice
Spirits
Stout malt liquor
Strawberry drinks
Sugar cane juice
Tanqueray
Tapioca drink coconut milk
Tea black
Tea caffeine
Tea decaffeinated
Tea green
Tea white
Tequila
Tequila methanol
Tomato juice
V8
Veg juice bottled canned BPA
Wine
Yogurt drinks with sugar animal milks

26. AVOID CHEMICALS

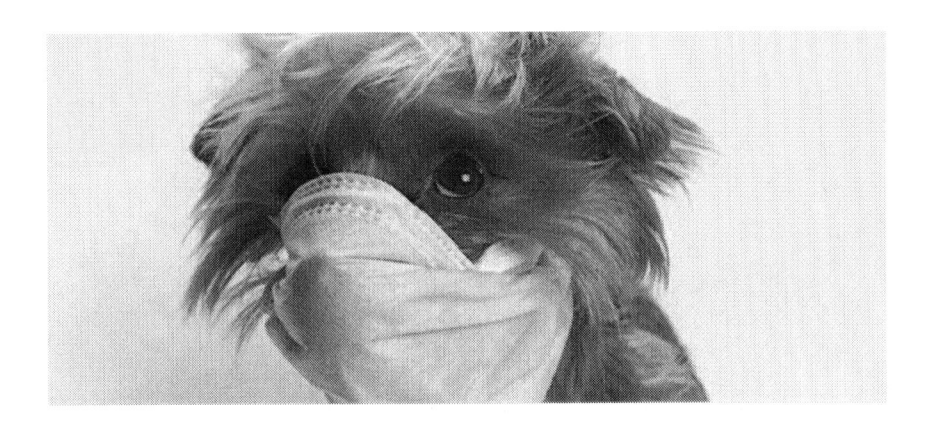

AVOID CHEMICALS

3-benzylidene-camphor
4-Methylbenzylidene sunscn
Acacia fiber
Acetaminophen
Acetylsalicylic acid
Acrylamide
ADA azodicarbonamide
Advil
Afinitor® Everolimus
Aflatoxin
Aging (NMN)
Air fresheners phthalates
Alcohol
Alcohol aerosol
Alcohol methanol

AVOID CHEMICALS

Aldomet

Aleve

Algae

Alkylphenols

Aluminum

Amalgam

Amino Acid L-arginine

Amino Acid L-canavanine

Amino Acid L-carnitine

Amiodarone

Ammonia

Anabolic steroids

Anti-inflammatory medication

Antifreeze

Apple hard cider

Arabitol

Aragonite all natural clay toothpaste

Arginine

Arsenic

Artificial sweetener

Aspartame (Nutrasweet)

Aspirin

Assugrin

Atrazine weed killer

Azodicarbonamide ADA

Baking soda taken regularly

AVOID CHEMICALS

Bathroom spray

BGH bovine growth hormone

BHA Butylated Hydroxyanisole

BHT Butylated hydroxytoluene

Bio-oil®

Birth control pills

Bisacodyl

Bisphenol A (BPA) plastic

Black seed oil

Blackstrap molasses

Bleach

Bleach cleanser

Blue-green algae

Botanique toothpaste

Bottled juices methanol

Bovine growth hormone

Braggs apple cider vinegar

Braggs liquid aminos

Brake fluid

Brown sugar

Bud-nip

Butter

ButylatedHydroxyanisole BHA

Cadmium

Caffeine

cAMP

AVOID CHEMICALS

Canavanine
Canned food ↑ methanol
Canned soups ↑ methanol
Canola oil
Carbamazepine (tegretol)
Carbon tetrachloride
Carnitine
Carrageenan
Casein
Chaga mushroom tea powder
Chemicals ↑ cough
Chlorella
Chloride
Chlorine comet
Chlorpropham
Chlorpyrifos
Chondroitin
Chowder with dairy
Cigarettes cigars chewing tobacco
Cimetidine
Cleanser with bleach
ClearLax
Clenz-Lyte
Clover honey
Co-Lav
Coconut ice cream carrageenan

AVOID CHEMICALS

Coconut oil

Colase®

Colax

Colchicine

Colchicum

Colgate toothpaste

Colovage

Colyte

Comet cleanser

Concentrated sugars

Constipation

Coral calcium

Coral white toothpaste

Cordarone (Amiodarone)

Cordyceps (fungi)

Cosmetics phenoxyethanol

Cosmetics with cod liver oil

Cottonseed oil caution aflatoxin

Crab

Cranberry pills

Cream

Cream cheese

Cream of tartar

Creamsicle

Creatine supplements

Crème fraîche

Crest toothpaste

AVOID CHEMICALS

Crisco
Cyclamate
Cyclic AMP
Daptacel vaccine (Phenoxyethanol)
DCA Dichloroacetate in tap water
DDD Dichlorodiphenyldichloroethane
DDE insecticide residue
DDT (dichlorodiphenyltrichloroethane)
DEHP PVC plasticizer
Detergents
Dichloroacetate DCA
Dichlorodiphenyldichloroethane
Dieldrin insecticide
Diethyl phthalate
Diethylstilbestrol
Diflucan
Doxidan
DPA Diphenylamine
DPT Diphenylthiazole
Dry cleaned clothing chemicals
Dryer sheets
Dulcolax
E-Z-Em Fortrans
Ecstasy
Eels
Endocrine disruptors
Endosulfan (insecticide)

AVOID CHEMICALS

Equal

Erythritol

Erythrosine FD C Red 3

Estrace

Estrogen

Estrogen BCP/pill/patch

Estrogen disruptors

Estrogenic shampoo

Ethanol

Ethylene glycol

Eugenol (oil cloves)

Everolimus

Excedrin

Fabric softener

Face cream

Famotidine

Fats

Fire retardants

Flagyl

Flaxseed oil capsules

Flounder

Fluconazole

Fluoride

Fontina cheese

Foods heated in plastic

Formaldehyde

Forskolin

AVOID CHEMICALS
Fragrance
Fragrance: BHT endocrine disruptor
Fragrance: Diethyl phthalate ~ hormone
Fragrance: Limonene → formaldehyde
Fragrance: Octinoxate endo disruptor
Fragrance: Oxybenzone endo disruptor
Fried foods
Fructose
Galactitol
Ganoderma lucidum
GaviLax
Gavilyte
Gelato
Genistein (soy)
Gentamicin
Germanium
Glucosamine
Glycolax
Glycols polyethylene → polyester
GlycoPrep
Glyphosate
GMO genetically modified
GMO seed
Go-Evac
GoLYTELY®
Grapeseed oil
Hair chemicals dye

AVOID CHEMICALS

Hair gel
HalfLytely
Heating food in microwave
Heptachlor (insecticide)
Herbicides
Homocysteine
Hormones
HRT Hormones
Hydrogenated starch hydrolysate HSH
Hydrolyzed wheat protein
Ibuprofen
Imitrex
Inflammatory foods
Jason Oral comfort toothpaste
Jason PowerSmile toothpaste
Ketoconazole
Kidney avoid
Kiss my face toothpaste
Kombucha
L-arginine
L-canavanine
L-carnitine
L'oreal HiP High Intensity Pigments
Lactitol
Laundry powder
Lax-a-Day
Laxatives

AVOID CHEMICALS
LaxLyte
Lead
Lecithin (soy)
Lectin
Limonene → formaldehyde
Lindane (insecticide)
Linseed oil
Liquid aminos
Lithium
Liver toxic
Lysergic Acid LSD
LytePrep
Macrogol
Magnesium
Margarine
Mederma scar cream
Menaquinone with soy
Mercury
Metalloestrogens
Methanol
Methanol alcoholic drinks
Methionine
Methoxychlor (insecticide)
Methyldopa
Methylisothiazolinone DNA damage
Methylparabens
Microwaved foods
Migraine

AVOID CHEMICALS
MiraLAX
MIT Methylisothiazolinone
MK-7 with soy
Motrin
Movicol
MoviPrep
MSG (monosodium glutamate)
MSM (methylsulfonylmethane)
Multiple vitamins
Nail chemicals polish removers
Naltrexone
Naproxen
Nattokinase
Natural dentist toothpaste
Natural tea tree toothpaste
Neatsfoot oil
Nectresse
Neem toothpaste
Neotame
Neutrogena body oil
Neutrogena facial cleanser
Niacin
Nicotinamide
Nitrites
Nitrosamine
Nizoral
NNM (N-nitrosomorpholine)
Non-dairy creamer

AVOID CHEMICALS

Non-stick teflon
Nonylphenol
Norbu
NSAIDs
NuLYTELY
Nutribiotic toothpaste
Nutritional yeast
OCL (laxative)
Octinoxate sunscreen
Oil canola
Oil coconut
Oil cottonseed
Oil grapeseed
Oil lavender
Oil palm
Oil sesame
Oil sunflower
Oil tea tree
Oils
Oilseeds caution aflatoxin
Olay daily facial cleaning cloth
Organic chlorinated pesticides
Organophosphorus pesticides
Ospemifene
Osphena™
Oven cleaners
Oxybenzone
PAH Polycyclic arom hydrocarbon

AVOID CHEMICALS
Palm oil
Paraben (lotion)
Paracetamol
PEG
Peg Lyte
Pentachlorophenol
Pepcid
Perchlorate
Perfluorinated Chemicals PFC
Perfume
PerioBrite toothpaste
Pesticides
Phenacetin
Phenol nonylphenol
Phenosulfothiazine red dye
Phenoxyethanol
Phthalates
Phytates phytic acid
Phytoestrogens i.e. soy
Pioglitazone (wait)
Plastic
Plastic wrap
Plexxicon PLX5568
Polychlorinated biphenyls
Polycyclic arom hydrocarbon PAH
Polyester
Polyethylene glycol
Pregnancy

AVOID CHEMICALS
Premarin
Prempro
Prep lyte
Processed foods
Progesterone (& creams)
PUFA Polyunsaturated fatty acids
Purelax
PureVia
PVC polyvinyl chloride
Ractopamine
Rapadura
Rapamune
Rapamycin
Red dye
Red yeast rice
Remifemin
Restore toothpaste
Resveratrol
Reversin
Revlon ColorStay Bronzer for the Face
Rolly toothpaste brush
Roscovitine
Roundup®
S-adensylmethionine
SAMe
Scar oil
Scent fragrance

AVOID CHEMICALS

Seliciclib

Shampoo with formaldehyde

Shampoo with methylisothiazolinone MIT

Shampoo with methylparabens

Shampoo with parabens

Shampoo with phthalates

Shampoo with sodium lauryl sulfate

Silver amalgam

Sirolimus

Soap powder

Sodium bicarbonate frequently

Sodium lauryl sulfate

Softlax

Solvent

Sorbitol (maltitol)

Soy lecithin

Soy sauce

Spiker water resistant styling glue

Spirits

Spirulina

Spray cleaners

Statins

Stem cells wait

Styrofoam containers

Sunflower oil

Sunscreen 4-Methylbenzylidene

Sunscreen benzophenone-3

AVOID CHEMICALS

Table sugar
Tacos
Tagamet
Tagatose sugar
Tamari
Tanqueray
Tea tree oils
Teeth plastic fillings
Teflon
Teriyaki sauce
Tesevatinib
Testosterone
Thymoquinone
Tilapia
Tilefish
TMAO Trimethylamine *N*-oxide
Tobacco
Tom's toothpaste
Trehalose (mycose)
Triclosan in water supply
TriLyte
Tylenol
Vegemite
Vinegar
Vitamin B3
Vitamin K2 with soy
Vytorin
Weed killer

AVOID CHEMICALS
Wild yam progesterone cream
Windex
Window cleaners
Worcestershire sauce
Xagave
Xanthan
Xenoestrogens
Xylitol spry toothpaste
Yeast

27. AVOID VEGETABLES

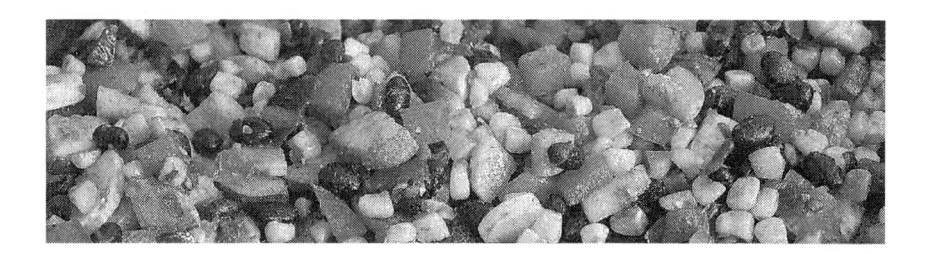

AVOID VEGETABLES
Agave cactus
Alfalfa sprouts
Aubergine
Auricularia polytricha (black fungus)
Baked potato
Bell peppers
Black fungus
Brinjal eggplant
Canned vegetables ↑ methanol
Capers
Capsicum annuum
Carrots dipped in bleach
Catchweed
Celery

AVOID VEGETABLES
Chilies
Cleaver
Cloud ear fungus
Clover sprouts
Corn if GMO
Dandelion greens
Dashi / Dill pickles
Edamame
Eggplant
French fries
Fried vegetables
Galium aparine (cleavers)
Ganoderma lucidum (lingzhi)
Glechoma hederacea (ivy)
Gold yukon potato
Goosegrass
Graviola soursop
Ground Ivy
Guarana

AVOID VEGETABLES

Hash browns

Iceberg lettuce

Jalapeño peppers

Lingzhi

Nattō from soy

Nightshade plants

Paprika

Peppers

Pickles

Pimenta dioica

Pimento

Potato

Potato chips

Precut vegetables

Produce dipped in bleach

Ready to eat vegetables

Red pimento

Red reishi

Red white potato

Reishi

AVOID VEGETABLES

Russet potato
Sea asparagus
Seaweed
Sorrel
Soursop
Soybeans
Spaghetti sauce
Spinach
Sprouts alfalfa
Sprouts clover
Sprouts soy
Sugar beets if GMO
Tannia leaf
Tomato
Tomatoes canned BHT methanol
Vegemite
Vichyssoise
Wild yam

AVOID VEGETABLES
Wild yam
Wood ear fungus
Yucca
Zucchini if GMO

28. AVOID FRUITS

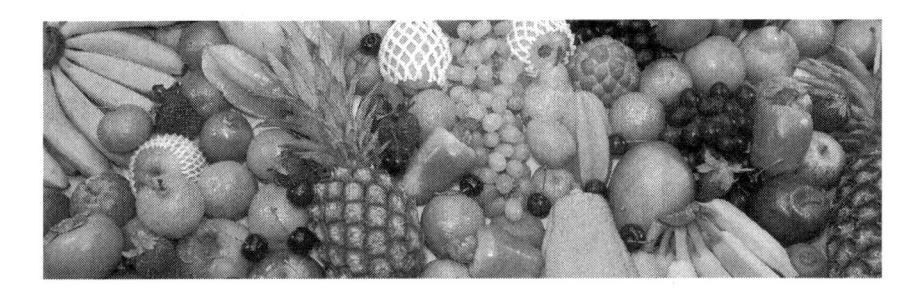

AVOID FRUITS
Açai
Ackee
Aronia melancarpa chokeberry
Averrhoa carambola
Bearberry whole fruit
Bilberry whole fruit
Blueberry whole fruit
Canned fruit ↑ methanol
Cantaloupe fungus transported
Cape gooseberry (poha)
Carambola
Chocolate dipped strawberry
Chokeberry whole fruit
Cranberry whole fruit
Dried fruit caution aflatoxin

AVOID FRUITS
Dried plum
Dried prune
Dried strawberry
Elderberry whole fruit
Fruit caution
Fruit dried caution aflatoxin
Garcinia cambogia (tamarind)
Goji berries
Grapefruit caution
Huckleberry whole fruit
L'amour encage
Lanzones
Longan
Lychee
Maraschino cherry
Melon transported develop fungus
Mountain apple
Mulberry whole fruit
Noni fruit
Pepino
Physalis peruviana (poha)
Plum

AVOID FRUITS
Poha berry
Pomegranate caution
Prickly pear
Prune
Rambutan
Rhubarb
Soursop
Starfruit
Strawberry
Sugar cane
Tamarind
Tropical mountain apples
Wax jambu (mountain apple)
Wolfberry (goji)

29. AVOID SWEETENERS

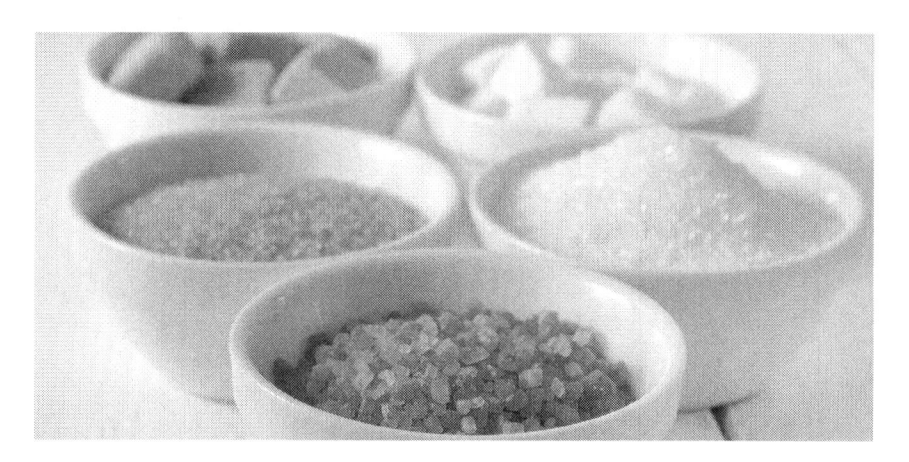

AVOID SWEETENERS
Acesulfame potassium
Agave Syrup
Almond dream ice cream
Almond ice cream with carrageenan
Arabitol
Artificial sweetener
Aspartame (Nutrasweet)
Assugrin
Banana split
Beet sugar
Blackstrap molasses
Brown rice syrup ↑ arsenic
Brown sugar
Candy

AVOID SWEETENERS
Cane juice crystals
Cane sugar
Caramels
Chitosan
Chocolate truffles
Chocolates
Clover honey
Coconut sugar
Concentrated sugar
Corn syrup
Cyclamate
Dark chocolate
Demerara sugar
Dessert
Dextrose
Equal
Erythritol
Fructose
Fudge
Galactitol
Hershey bars
HFCS
High fructose corn syrup HFCS
Hydrogenated starch hydrolysate HSH
Isomalt
Jaggery

AVOID SWEETENERS

Just like sugar
Lactitol
Lesys (Maltitol, maltisweet, sweetPearl)
Lollipop
Maltisweet (Maltitol Lesys SweetPearl)
Maltitol
Mannitol
Maple syrup
Molasses
Monk fruit in the raw sweetener (contains dextrose)
Muscovado sugar
Mycose
Nectresse
Neotame
Norbu
NutraSweet (aspartame)
Panela
Peanut butter cups
Pearl sweet
Piloncillo
Popsicle
Prune butter
PureVia
Red clover honey
Rice ice cream carrageenan
Rice syrup

AVOID SWEETENERS

Saccharin
Sorbitol (maltitol)
Splenda
Stevia
Sucanat
Sucralose
Sucrose
Sugar
Sugar cane crystals
Sugar twin
Sunett (asesulfame potassium, Ace-K)
Sweet One
Sweet'N Low
SweetPearl (maltitol)
Table sugar
Tagatose sugar
Trehalose (mycose)
Truvia
Turbinado sugar
White beet sugar
White cane sugar
White chocolate
Xagave
Xylitol

30. EVERYONE TO AVOID

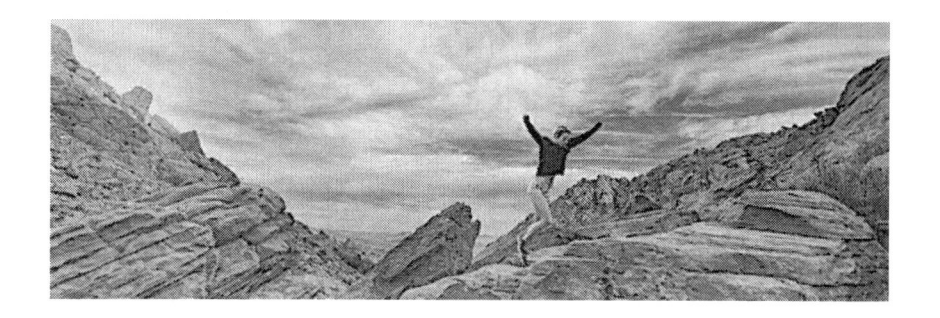

Aluminum

Artificial sweeteners

Candy

Crisco

French Fries

Lard

Margarine

Peanuts

Potato chips

Processed foods

White flour

White potato

White sugar

31. MENU

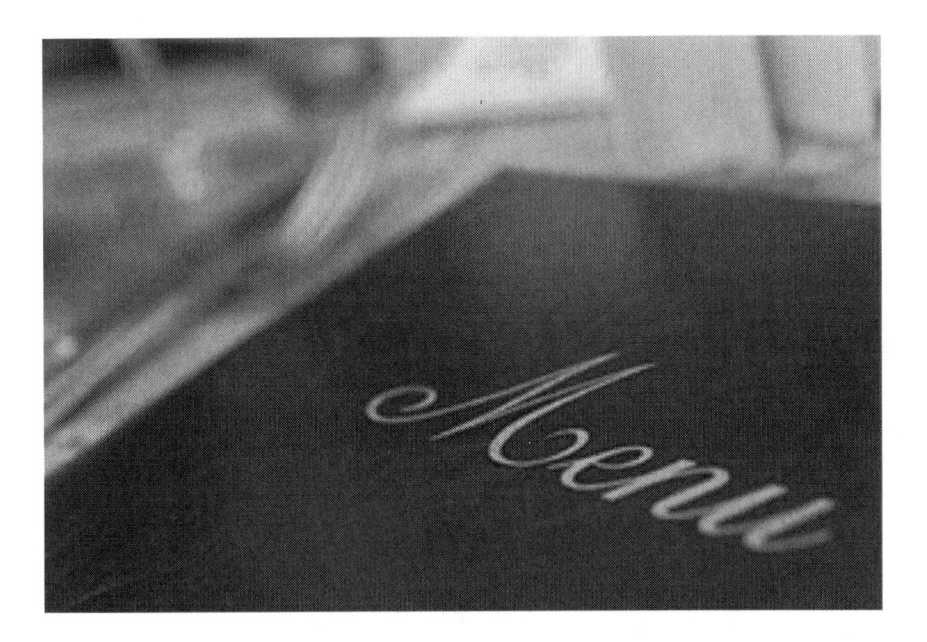

Upon Arising Menu

One teaspoon of solé in a glass of water.
After eating raw fruit or drinking citrus, please allow 20 minutes before taking something else.
Freshly squeezed lemon juice, add enough water to make ¼ cup.
Grapefruit juice freshly squeezed (caution interferes with many medications).
Allow 20 minutes before taking something else.
Throughout the day, if permitted, drink water equal to twice your output (or ~4Liters) thus turning off vasopressin, a hormone that stimulates cyst growth.

Breakfast Menu

After eating raw fruit or drinking citrus, allow 20 minutes before taking something else.

Fruit: Raw fresh fruit in season & locally grown: banana, figs, kiwi, kumquats, pear, grapefruit, apple, clementine or if in the tropics: mango, papaya, jack fruit (the biggest and one of the sweetest fruits in the world and it hangs ripening from a majestic tree), pomelo, cherimoya. During berry season a bowl filled with ripe red raspberries, black raspberries and blackberries from the wild might be a start for the day.

Strawberries are too acid forming & one of the highest fruits with pesticides, thus joining fruits to be avoided: starfruit, rhubarb, strawberry, plum, prunes, rambutan, poha berry, lychee, longan, ackee.

Fruit: Freshly sliced grapefruit (caution grapefruit interferes with certain medications).

Fruit: Bananas and apples or stewed fruit.

Fruit: Freshly squeezed orange juice.

Cereal: Corn meal with chopped dates. Soak grains overnight.

Cereal: Hot cereal made from spelt, rye, kamut, brown rice, grits, corn meal, steel cut oats or oatmeal with almond, coconut, hempseed, barley, oat, or rice milk.

Hot cereal: Prepare ½ cup of spelt kernels that have been soaked overnight to diminish phytic acid. Whole spelt kernels have a taste similar to a bowl of ground nuts. Grind the kernels in a food processor. The following morning heat and top with banana, dates, pears, or cinnamon apples.

Breakfast Menu

Toasted non-yeasted English Muffin spelt, rye, kamut, brown rice~caution ↑ arsenic, corn with an all fruit spread or almond butter or both.

Toasted non-yeasted non-wheat bread spelt, rye, kamut, brown rice~caution ↑ arsenic, corn with an all fruit spread or almond butter or both.

Toasted non-yeasted non-wheat bagel: spelt, rye, kamut, brown rice~caution ↑ arsenic, corn.

Warmed non-yeasted pita: spelt, rye, kamut, corn stuffed with chopped cilantro, garlic, and avocado.

Warmed non-yeasted Baps: spelt, rye, kamut, corn stuffed with chopped cilantro, garlic, and avocado.

Warmed non-yeasted pita: spelt, rye, kamut, corn stuffed with chopped cilantro garlic, and avocado.

Toasted non-yeasted non-wheat bread spelt, rye, kamut, brown rice, corn

with sautéed mushrooms, almond butter, cashew butter, bean spread, or avocado are a few alternative spreads.
Essene bread spread with almond butter.
Warmed corn tortillas; homemade spelt chapattis or another non-yeasted flat breads such as parathas, crackers, and spelt dosas. These taste so much better when freshly prepared by yourself without yeast.
Non-yeasted breads made with spelt, rye, kamut, corn, brown rice~caution ↑ arsenic: the dough is a flour and water mixture. This rises for 7 hours before baked. Unlike yeasted breads which rise quickly; non-yeasted breads release their digestive enzymes in the lactic acid ferment. This lactic acid can be blown off by several deep breaths throughout the day. Other acids produced by the body increase the workload upon cystic kidneys, this in turn affects the liver. After eating non-yeasted spelt bread many have noticed that they never come away with a bloated feeling. It is similar when soaking nuts, beans, legumes and seeds to lessen their phytic acid content. With large ever expanding cystic organs, it is very useful to minimize bloating. Many with liver cysts take H2 blockers. In theory this slows down secretin and prevents liver cysts from expanding.

Liquids

Liquids: enjoy following solid food. Eat a raw slice of alkaline fruit twenty minutes before a meal. After eating raw fruit or drinking citrus, please allow 20 minutes before taking something else.
Herb Tea Chamomile, chamomile citrus, hibiscus, lemon grass, lemon thyme, lemon water, linden flower, milk thistle, rose hips, saffron tea, silymarin, sugar cookie sleigh ride, thyme, tilleul, or veronica tea.
Roasted grain beverage: barley brew, barley cup, cafix, caro, carob powder, inka, java herb uncoffee, kara kara, organic instant grain, prewetts chicory, roma, spelt kaffee, or teeccino.
Water: Lemon water, mineral water, spring water or water that has been left out for 24 hours to dissipate any chlorine.

Morning Snack Menu

Fruit: 20 minutes before lunch have an alkaline fruit: apple, pear, kiwi, pineapple, cherries, grapes, banana or papaya.
Fruit: Dried apricot, raisins, mango without sugar, cherries, dates, apples. Caution check for mold and do not eat if any has developed as this can contain aflatoxin a known carcinogen..
Fruit: After eating raw fruit or citrus or their juices please allow 20 minutes before taking something else.

Juice: cabbage-almond, apple, beet-apple, kale-grape.
Juice: ¼ wedge of cabbage with 5-7 almonds enough to produce 2 ounces of juice.
Juice: 2 apples, half a lemon peeled, small slice of galangal (Thai ginger) ¼ beet.
Grains: Unsalted organic corn chips, brown rice cakes, unsalted spelt, rye, corn, rice pretzels or spelt, rye, corn, rice crackers. Caution with rice as it may contain some arsenic.
Nuts: Young coconut water and enjoy the coconut gelatin like spoon meat.
Nuts: Roasted chestnuts.
Nuts: (7) roasted almonds.
Smoothie: mixture of pineapple, banana, apple orange.
Vegetables: raw carrots, jicama, (5) radish, turnip.

Liquids

Enjoy liquids following eating solid food.
Herb Tea Chamomile, chamomile citrus, hibiscus, lemon grass, lemon thyme, lemon water, linden flower, milk thistle, rose hips, saffron tea, silymarin, sugar cookie sleigh ride, thyme, tilleul, or veronica tea.
Roasted grain beverage: barley brew, barley cup, cafix caro, carob powder, inka, java herb uncoffee, kara kara, organic instant grain, prewetts chicory, roma, spelt kaffee, teeccino.
Water: Lemon water, mineral water, spring water or water that has been left out for 24 hours to dissipate any chlorine.

Lunch Menu

Soup: Lentil or bean soup with brown rice. Caution rice may contain arsenic.
Soup: Coconut milk and vegetables with brown rice. Caution rice may contain arsenic.
Soup sides: spelt bread, spelt crackers, corn tortillas, brown rice crackers. Caution rice may contain arsenic.
Salad: romaine lettuce, sliced radish, diced carrot, purple onion, mushrooms, jicama, turnip (quick dip leafy greens in hot water or lemon to diminish oxalates).
Sandwich: Almond vegetable paté on non-yeasted spelt, kamut, or corn bread or as hor d'oeuvres this spread can be placed on a sliced cucumber or zucchini.
Sandwich: Vegetable burger made without soy or wheat on non-yeasted

spelt, kamut, or corn bread bun.
Sandwich: Almond butter and fruit spread or sliced banana.Lunch Menu
Sandwich: Pita with diced steamed vegetables (spelt, kamut, or corn pita).
Sandwich: Walnut vegetable paté lettuce, purple onion, cucumber.
Vegetables: Moroccan vegetable stew with beans.
Vegetables: Vegetables wrapped in a romaine lettuce leaf.
Vegetables: Buddha's delight.

Liquids

Enjoy liquids following eating solid food.
Herb Tea   Chamomile, chamomile citrus, chocolate hibiscus, lemon grass, lemon thyme, lemon water, linden flower, milk thistle, rose hips, saffron tea, silymarin, sugar cookie sleigh ride, thyme, tilleul, or veronica tea.
Roasted grain beverage: barley brew, barley cup, cafix, caro, carob powder, inka, java herb uncoffee, kara kara, organic instant grain, prewetts chicory, roma, spelt kaffee or teeccino.
Water: Lemon water, mineral water, spring water or water that has been left out for 24 hours to dissipate chlorine.

Dinner Menu

Raw spring roll with cubed carrots, onions, peas, radish, mint.
Pasta: spelt pasta fettuccine with roasted squash, chard, kale, almonds, garlic, lemon or spring onionsPie: Vegetable pie.
Pie: Wild mushroom shepherd's pie made with root vegetables.
Pizza spelt crust Ø yeast with mushrooms, onion, garlic.
Polenta crispy with roasted vegetables.
Vegetables: Roasted root vegetables: rutabagas, carrots, sweet potatoes, turnips, beets, and some above ground crops such as artichokes, carrots, or squash.
Vegetables: Steamed array of vegetables: corn, squash, onion, garlic, celeriac, pumpkin, sunchokes, artichokes.
Vegetables with brown rice~caution ↑ arsenic, squash risotto.
Vegetables: Vegetables with spelt pasta.
Vegetables: All vegetable Terrine or Paté
To diminish symptoms continue to avoid nightshade plants: tomatoes, bell peppers, eggplant, potatoes.
Vegetables: All vegetable tagine chickpeas, saffron, cilantro over quinoa.
Vegetables: Corn cakes with walnut sauce, braised oxblood carrots with spelt pasta.

Vegetables: Mushroom tart with leeks.
Vegetables: Curries cauliflower and peas with brown rice. Caution rice ↑ arsenic.
Vegetables: Moroccan vegetable curry.
Vegetables: Slow roasted Okinawan sweet potatoes; braised carrots; steamed corn; sautéed leafy greens with currants, garlic, lemon.
Vegetables: Brown rice~caution ↑ arsenic, and beans.
Vegetables: Pot-au-feu made of all vegetables.

Liquids

Liquids: Enjoy liquids after solid food: a cup of herb tea, nettle extract in warm water; thyme tea; veronica tea; grain beverage or water.

Late Night Snack

Water: Place water by the bed with a lemon slice if desired.
Juice: Grape juice (all juice) with 2 ounces of mineral water.
Juice: Cranberry (all juice) with 2 ounces of mineral water. If urine is too alkaline in the evening, cranberry juice will make it slightly more acidic.
Herb Tea Chamomile tea with tupelo honey if desired.
Herb Tea Saffron tea made without any honey.

32. HELPFUL WEBSITES

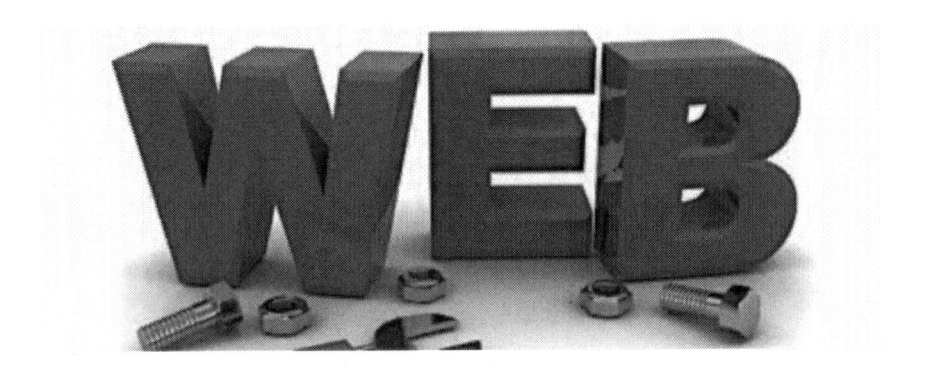

CYSTIC ORGANS
http://www.CysticOrgan.com

KIDNEY
http://www.polycystic-kidneydisease.com/index2.html

LIVER
http://www.polycysticliverdisease.com/index2.html

PKD RECIPE INSPIRATIONS
http://www.pkdrecipes.com

PKD DETAILS
http://www.pkdiet.com/index2.php

ALKALINE DIET
http://www.alkalinediet.com/enjoy.html

33. DERMATOLOGY SYMPTOMS

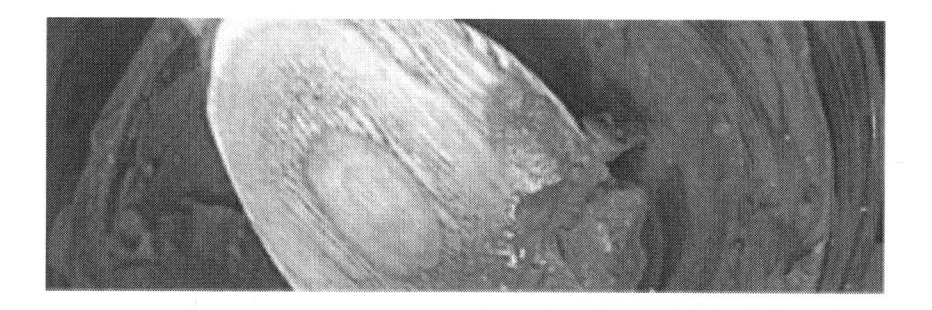

Sometimes we get itchy skin, thinning hair, whitened nails, cramping legs. Many personal care products aggravate PKD Polycystic Kidney symptoms or increase cyst growth. EWG has a database rating of many personal products.

To diminish itching try using bentonite clay paste in lieu of soap. While in the shower, apply olive oil on the skin. Then under running water, rub on bentonite clay paste (recipe follows). Wrap a sliced lemon in cheese cloth. Gently rub the cut surface of the wrapped lemon over the skin. Apply additional olive oil; rinse with water. Sprinkle baking soda on wet skin to help remove any residual oil; a final rinse with copious amounts of water; then pat dry. These methods help ease itching and dry skin.

BENTONITE RECIPE

1 cup of clay
1 cup of olive oil, add sufficient to make a paste
1 teaspoon of tupelo honey

Some have tried eliminating shampoo and using a clay hair masque.

RHASSOUL RECIPE

Rhassoul (Ghassoul) Moroccan clay hair masque
Black rubber bowl used to mix plaster (3 cup size)
2 Tablespoons of red Moroccan clay
1-2 drops of burdock oil (Klettenwurzel Haar-Oil)
Wire whisk
Warm water

CAUTION olive oil can make shower surfaces very slippery.

Mix together forming a paste. Apply on damp hair. Leave on for about an hour. Then rinse. A few more suggestions are available.

Some other things a few PKD'rs have found helpful: clay baths, saunas, eating: radishes, DIMs (broccoli sprouts), sunchokes and cabbage. If the day ever arrives when kidney functioning becomes diminished, taking clay baths is one possibility that takes advantage of the entire skin surface as an additional organ to help diminish body toxins. Saunas allow the body's sweat to help lower kidney toxins. Cabbage juice, turmeric, and DIMs (broccoli sprouts) encourage the metabolism of any endocrine disruptors throughout the body by increasing estrogen metabolism through the liver. Radishes help raise the ecoplast of the red blood cells and help with anemia.

34. ALKALINE CLINICAL TRIALS

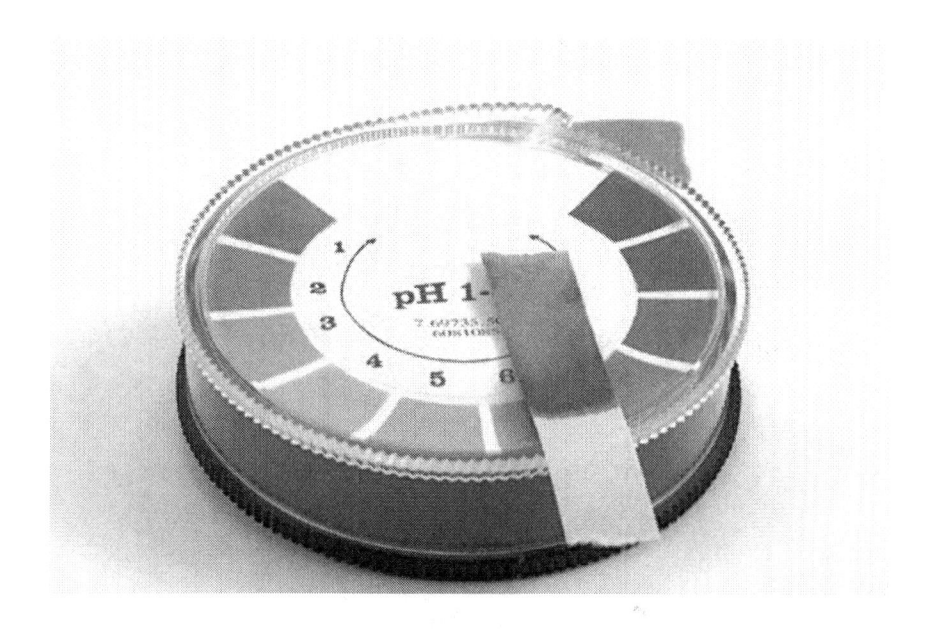

The time may be ideal for an Alkaline PKD Clinical Trial. 1998 PKD research by the Tanners showed Citrate Therapy improved PKD renal functioning:

http://www.pkdiet.com/pdf/kcitanner/kcit1998.pdf.

In 2000 research showed that Citrate therapy or alkalinity improved PKD.

http://www.pkdiet.com/pdf/kcitanner/kcit2000.pdf

ALKALINE CLINICAL TRIALS

http://www.polycysticliverdisease.com/pdf/AlkalineTrial.pdf

2010 Clinical Trial sodium citrate-alkalinity improves GFR
https://www.ncbi.nlm.nih.gov/pubmed/20072112

2010 Clinical Trial completed using potassium citrate in renal transplant patients
https://clinicaltrials.gov/ct2/show/NCT00913796

2010 Basic approach to chronic kidney disease
https://www.ncbi.nlm.nih.gov/pubmed/20224583

2010 Alkaline Diet reduces urinary oxalate excretion, prominent in PKD
https://www.ncbi.nlm.nih.gov/pubmed/20736987

2010 Urinary alkalization for the treatment of uric acid
https://www.ncbi.nlm.nih.gov/pubmed/21121431

2010 Clinical Trial potassium citrate boosts bone density in the elderly
http://www.polycystic-kidneydisease.com/pdf/BoneDensity.pdf

2010 Veggie diet best for kidney patients
http://www.medpagetoday.com/Nephrology/GeneralNephrology/24060

2010 Clinical Trial: acid retention leads to progressive GFR decline, remedied by alkaline diet
https://www.ncbi.nlm.nih.gov/pubmed/20861823

2013 Clinical Trial: plant based protects against renal toxicity and loss of DNA integrity
http://www.pkdiet.com/pdf/AlkalineTrial/PlantBasedDiet.pdf

2014 Plant Based MultiCenter Study Reduces Depression Anxiety & Improves Quality of Life
https://www.ncbi.nlm.nih.gov/pubmed/24524383

2014 Dietary Patterns Risk of Death Progression ESRD in Individuals with CKD: A Cohort
https://www.ncbi.nlm.nih.gov/pubmed/24679894

2014 Plant Based Diet Lowers Risk of Renal Cell Carcinoma in Large US Cohort Study
http://www.pkdiet.com/pdf/AlkalineTrial/PlantFoodsRCC.pdf

2016 Food Restriction Ameliorates Development of PKD
https://www.ncbi.nlm.nih.gov/pubmed/26538633

2016 Fatty Acid Impaired in PKD Model
https://www.ncbi.nlm.nih.gov/pubmed/27077126

2017 Dietary Salt Restriction Beneficial PKD
https://www.ncbi.nlm.nih.gov/pubmed/27993381

35. THE FUTURE

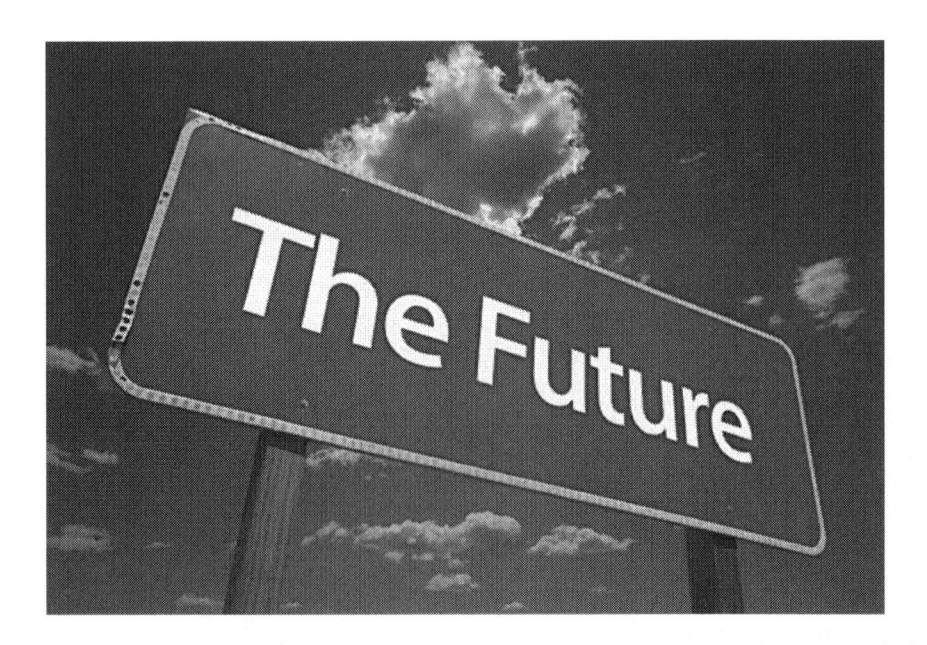

We are hopeful and optimistic that in the foreseeable future a PKD Diet will become commonplace as an adjunctive medical therapy for PKD; its utilization will become as clear-cut as incorporating a diabetic diet in the treatment of diabetes.

Clinging to the prospect that conceivably what may lie ahead for us is a home unit with the ability for testing of our electrolytes and alkalinity (similar to existing home blood sugar kits). We imagine that the existence of such a machine could be coupled with the PKD Diet, bringing about true alkalinity and health for many with cystic organ disease.

No one is sure why alkalinity works for PKD. Our personal experience is that it is indeed helpful. A determination can be made through a clinical trial. Together, let us begin PKD alkaline trials. Let us dream about a bright PKD future.